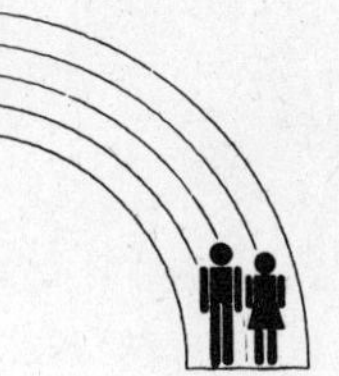

HIGH
BLOOD
PRESSURE

HELP YOURSELF TO HEALTH

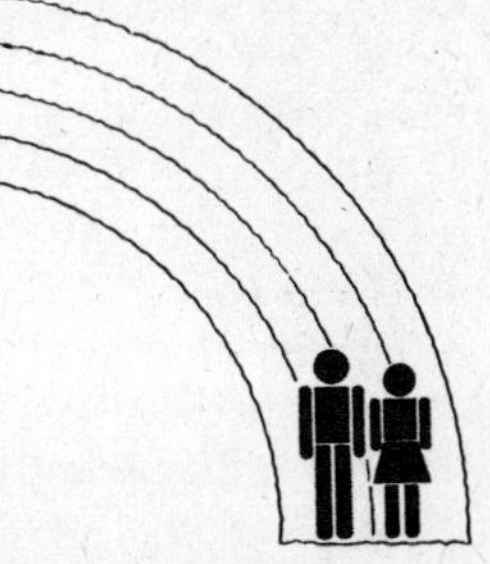

HIGH BLOOD PRESSURE

ADA P. KAHN, M.P.H.

Contemporary Books, Inc.
Chicago

Library of Congress Cataloging in Publication Data

Kahn, Ada P.
   High blood pressure.

   (Help yourself to health)
   Includes index.
      1. Hypertension—Addresses, essays, lectures.
I. Title.   II. Series: Help yourself to health series.
RC685.H8K34   1983   616.1'32   83-1969
 ISBN 0-8092-5599-5

Published by Contemporary Books, Inc.
180 North Michigan Avenue, Chicago, Illinois 60601
Manufactured in the United States of America
Library of Congress Catalog Card Number: 83-1969
International Standard Book Number: 0-8092-5599-5

Published simultaneously in Canada by
Beaverbooks, Ltd.
150 Lesmill Road
Don Mills, Ontario M3B 2T5
Canada

Contents

Foreword

We have known for a long time that uncontrolled high blood pressure is a serious health hazard and an important contributing cause of heart failure, kidney failure, and strokes—conditions that are among the leading causes of death in this country. Earlier than 15–20 years ago many physicians tended to be apathetic about high blood pressure in spite of this knowledge, probably because the basis of the condition was not well understood and the means to manage it were unreliable or difficult for patients to follow.

In more than 90 percent of all cases of high blood pressure no single cause is clearly identifiable. But newer, better tolerated drugs and a fuller appreciation of the value of moderation in consumption of salt, control of obesity, and avoidance of smoking have stimulated a more aggressive attitude toward detection and treatment of this serious health threat on the part of both physicians and the public at large. A very important factor in this new attitude has been the clear demonstration in several studies, done over a period of years and involving thousands of patients, that high blood pressure greatly increases the risk of cardiovascular disability and death. Other studies proved that individuals whose high blood pressure was treated properly, including those with mild high blood pressure, showed a great improvement in long-term health and life expectancy. The mortality rate from coronary artery disease in the United States has declined steadily since 1970. Many experts believe that more effective and widely used treatment of hypertension and the reduction of other risk factors for cardiovascular disease have played an important role in this exciting improvement in our nation's health.

The serious effects of uncontrolled high blood pressure have been all too frequently apparent in my 30-plus years of private clinical practice in internal medicine. During the last two decades I have also monitored the work of other physicians in an active union management health program of which I am medical director. Here I have seen many additional instances of the threats to health and longevity posed by high blood pressure and the impressive benefits that can be achieved through proper management of the condition. In this endeavor patient understanding and active cooperation are essential.

This excellent book by Ada P. Kahn, MPH, a writer who has worked in the field of health education for more than 25 years, fills a real need in bringing before the public optimistic, practical information about high blood pressure and how patients and their families can take full advantage of medical advice and treatment in controlling the disease.

The author has full command of the facts about high blood pressure and its management. The book is written in a clear, upbeat style that facilitates the reader's comprehension of the complex factors leading to high blood pressure and how the patient can improve his or her long-term health and well-being through relatively simple changes in lifestyle and by paying attention to medical advice.

This book should have wide appeal to interested lay persons and enjoy repeated use as a practical home reference source about high blood pressure and associated cardiovascular problems.

Robert B. Burton, MD, FACP

Acknowledgments

The author thanks Robert B. Burton, MD, for his assistance in making editorial changes to clarify some of the technical explanations in this manuscript. His cooperation has contributed greatly to the readability of the book.

Thanks also to the Chicago Heart Association and the American Heart Association for making current reference materials available and to the Department of Hypertension and Nephrology, The Cleveland Clinic, Cleveland, Ohio, for permitting several charts and tables to be used in this book.

Research assistants Ruth D. Kahn and Michael Kite provided valuable assistance.

Finally, the author thanks Jeremiah Stamler, MD, Chairman, Department of Community Health and Preventive Medicine, School of Medicine, Northwestern University, Chicago, Illinois, for his encouragement.

Introduction

If you have been told that you have hypertension (high blood pressure), you probably have many questions about preserving your good health. Whether you are new in the ranks of the 60 million Americans who have high blood pressure or have had it for a long time, this book will tell you what you should know about high blood presure and what you can do for yourself to bring it under control.

This book will help you understand what blood pressure is all about, what "high" or "low" blood pressure means, and why careful attention to your blood pressure and your physician's recommendations is so important to your continued good health. Also, this book will give you a foundation of information from which you can better understand and follow your physician's instructions for controlling your high blood pressure.

There are several things you can do right now to preserve your good health. By changing your diet, adding exercise to your lifestyle, stopping smoking, reducing your intake of alcoholic beverages and following other recommendations your physician will make, you can prevent complications that might endanger your good health.

Good health is your most precious possession. Yet, like most of us, you probably think more about trying to regain it when it may be lost than about protecting it while you are well. We purchase "sickness" or "hospitalization" insurance to help pay bills while we recover from illness or injury. Such insurance pays off only if we are ill. Insurance against high blood pressure isn't available. You have to be your own insurer. This book will help you learn how to control what experts say is the current single greatest hazard to good health: high blood pressure. You can take charge now by beginning a healthier daily routine—one which you will like.

As your insurance manual, this book will tell you what you should know to guard your precious possession, health, or perhaps the health of someone you love. It will tell you about your body's internal equipment relating to your blood pressure, how it works, why things sometimes go wrong, what to do as regular maintenance, and what to do in case of real trouble.

To encourage you to maintain the aspects of your body's mechanisms that affect blood pressure, you will learn about your heart and circulatory system; the importance of diet, exercise, and lifestyle; and how you can benefit from research studies. With this information you can take actions to help your physician control your high blood pressure so that you can enjoy a more productive life.

You can benefit right away from recent advances in research by understanding the importance of high blood pressure as a contributing factor in other diseases. During the past few years researchers have made significant advances in studying high blood pressure. They are sure that high blood pressure is a major contributor to various forms of heart and kidney disease. They now know that previously used terms, such as *borderline* and *mild* high blood pressure, are dangerous and misleading. Blood pressure in this so-called borderline area is now regarded as a significant risk factor for future disease. Researchers who have studied high blood pressure know that it is a predictor of future potential for illness, disability, or reduced life expectancy. Because of this evidence, many physicians have changed their attitudes about treating "mild" high blood pressure. They have moved from what some have called "therapeutic nihilism" (doing nothing) to taking positive steps to reduce blood pressure through appropriate medical care and behavioral changes that include diet and weight loss, exercise, cessation of smoking, and moderation of alcohol use. Research studies have shown that the possibilities for controlling your high blood pressure and preventing other diseases are good. By following these positive steps you have the opportunity to help yourself to continued good health.

As an introductory or refresher handbook, this book will give you some ideas for questions to ask your doctor regarding control of your high blood pressure. You'll be able to expand your high blood pressure vocabulary because medical terminology is explained. You will learn to use terms accurately and be able to discuss the importance of controlling high blood pressure with someone you love who hasn't read the book. A glossary has been included at the back of the book to define some words in more detail.

Now you are ready to start working as your own insurer. You will find helpful information you can use to control your high blood pressure, protect yourself against complications, and reduce the possibilities of premature disability—or death—from a preventable cause.

HELP YOURSELF TO HEALTH

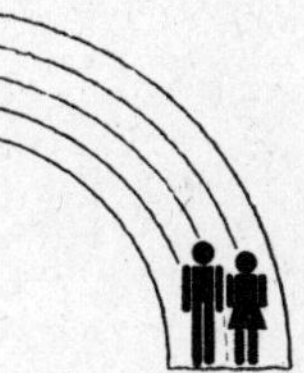

HIGH BLOOD PRESSURE

1

Getting Acquainted with High Blood Pressure

You've been told that you have high blood pressure. Why you? You thought you were a healthy person. Does having high blood pressure mean you're not healthy? What does having high blood pressure mean for your future health? What should you do now? What *can* you do?

High blood pressure can affect any of us. People of all ages can have it, even babies and young children. High blood pressure often runs in families, and a child or sibling of someone who has it runs an increased risk of having it. You're not alone with your high blood pressure. According to the High Blood Pressure Information Center of the National Institutes of Health, 60 million Americans have it. That's about one out of every four of us. While high blood pressure is the most common of the diseases affecting the heart and blood vessels, it is perhaps the most treatable, especially if detected in its early stages.

High blood pressure is not something that will just go away if you forget about it. It must and can be treated effectively. It is important to have appropriate treatment and to follow your doctor's instructions. Doing so may help you prevent a heart attack, stroke, or kidney disease. Following the treatment plan tailored to your needs can enable you to continue to lead a happy and productive life.

HOW THIS BOOK CAN HELP YOU

Because you are a unique individual, the precise factors that led to your high blood pressure may be a little different from those that caused your friend's or neighbor's. Each person has his or her own package of hereditary factors and personal habits. The ways you eat, exercise, and live each day interact and may determine whether you develop high blood pressure. This book will help you understand how your own lifestyle may have contributed to your high blood pressure and how altering it can help you control your high blood pressure.

Your physician will design your treatment plan to fit the personal package that may have led to your high blood pressure. For example, your high blood pressure may be of the type that responds well to changes in dietary habits, such as reducing or eliminating salt from the diet and moderating intake of alcohol and caffeine, and in exercise habits. Such lifestyle changes work well for many people. In other cases medications are needed to bring high blood pressure under control. Medication for high blood pressure differs among individuals. Doses of high blood pressure medications are always tailored to fit individual needs. Most people with high blood pressure who are treated through changes in lifestyle, through medication, or both, have a normal life expectancy. Treatment is important, however, because untreated high blood pressure is a major risk factor for complications such as heart and kidney disease. How well you follow your doctor's plan for your treatment will determine its success. This book will help you understand your doctor's recommendations and the reasons for them.

THE IMPORTANCE OF CONTROLLING HIGH BLOOD PRESSURE

Controlling high blood pressure is important because of the seriousness of the complications that may result when high blood pressure is untreated. Blood pressure is the amount of force required to circulate your blood throughout your body. High blood pressure makes your heart and blood vessels work harder and can lead to several major diseases. Heart disease is one. The extra strain on your heart can cause the walls of your heart to thicken and become damaged. You'll learn more about your circulatory system and how high blood pressure affects your heart in Chapter 2.

High blood pressure can also strain your blood vessels too much, so that they become narrowed and lose their ability to stretch. When a blood vessel in the brain becomes sufficiently weakened or narrowed and finally ruptures or obstructs, a stroke (cerebrovascular accident) can occur. Varying degrees of paralysis or loss or mental function can result from strokes.

Kidney disease is a third possible result of high blood pressure. The tiny arteries in the kidneys are damaged by the excessive pressure. After enough damage the kidneys stop filtering out waste products, and illness can follow. You'll learn more about the possible complications you are trying to avoid in Chapter 5.

WHAT CAN YOU DO?

Your high blood pressure may have been detected during a visit to your dentist's office, at a community health center, or elsewhere. Now that you know you have it, you should take steps to reduce it and preserve your good health.

Your first step will be to consult a physician, if you have not already done do. Your doctor will explain high blood pressure and its relationship to heart disease. No one single factor is responsible for causing heart disease; many causes interrelate. But your physician will emphasize that high blood pressure is the most important single factor. When coupled with elevated blood fat levels, cigarette smoking, high salt intake, possibly diabetes, and perhaps high coffee and alcohol intake, high blood pressure can contribute to heart disease. You can alter many of these factors in an effort to prevent serious consequences. You can prevent the harmful effects of high blood pressure by having it measured regularly, by paying attention to your physician's advice, and by taking any prescribed medication.

When your physician outlines a treatment plan it is important to follow it carefully. Be receptive to suggestions for changes in your lifestyle. The changes won't affect just your high blood pressure; they will contribute to better health overall. If your doctor recommends medications, be sure to take them as prescribed, even if you have no symptoms. You may be like many who have high blood pressure and have no symptoms. Many people live for years without knowing they have it. High blood pressure usually gives no warning. It can be detected only by using a blood pressure gauge.

WHAT YOUR PHYSICIAN CAN DO

During early visits your physician will ask many questions about your habits and daily routines. Are you overweight? What do you eat? Do you eat a lot of fatty or salty foods? Do you exercise regularly? Are you active or sedentary in your job? Do you get adequate relaxation each day? From your responses your physician may recommend that you lose weight, eat fewer fatty and salty foods, and exercise more. Your doctor may recommend a medication to help reduce your blood pressure. You'll learn more about various high blood pressure medications in Chapter 8.

Your physician will measure your blood pressure during each visit with a special device that is explained in Chapter 2. You may be advised to monitor your blood pressure at home. How that is done is detailed in Chapter 9.

HOW DOCTORS VIEW HIGH BLOOD PRESSURE

Physicians agree that early attention to high blood pressure, especially before it is severely elevated, may make your life healthier and longer. They now emphasize that control of high blood pressure through early detection and treatment can prevent further threats to good health. The current attitude of physicians regarding blood pressure stems from findings of carefully controlled studies, which confirmed that those who have high blood pressure are more likely to develop other cardiovascular diseases than those with normal blood pressure, something life insurance companies have known for many years.

Until recently physicians noted that some patients had so-called "borderline" high blood pressure and used terms such as *mild* and *benign* to describe the condition. There is evidence now that even slightly elevated blood pressure may indicate the risk of future illness.

A dramatic statement from heart research authorities came in 1982 when the National High Blood Pressure Education Program of the National Heart, Lung and Blood Institute issued a warning that mild high blood pressure should no longer be considered mild. Results from a five-year national study showed that early treatment of what used to be called "mild" high blood pressure could save many lives. The study, the Hypertension Detection and Followup Program, showed that even mild high blood pressure can damage the cardiovascular system and the kidneys. If left untreated, mild high blood pressure can rise even higher and can cause a stroke, a heart attack, or kidney problems.

In the next chapters you'll learn ways of measuring blood pressure and better understand the importance of this study.

A diastolic pressure (see Glossary) of 90–103 mm Hg (millimeters of mercury) was considered mild high blood pressure. But according to these findings, those who have high blood pressure above 89 mm Hg diastolic are subject to twice the cardiovascular risk of individuals with readings below that figure.

Until this report most physicians treated only those with high blood pressure *above* the so-called mild range. The new information has caused physicians to redefine *high blood pressure* and has led them to treat it earlier with recommendations for changes in dietary and exercise habits and, in many cases, with one of several effective drugs.

Doctors say the best way to prevent complications of high blood pressure is to control several factors that contribute to it. These factors include being overweight, smoking, and consuming large amounts of salt, alcohol, and possibly caffeinated beverages. The ways in which you can reduce these factors in your life and reduce your blood pressure will be detailed in the following chapters.

HELPING YOURSELF

If you or someone about whom you care has ever been told to "watch your blood pressure," it may be time to have it checked again. If you were once in the so-called mild high blood pressure category, new information makes it imperative for you to have it checked and follow your physician's advice to keep it under control.

Only you can make sure your treatment plan is carried out properly, so take responsibility in improving your own health. Stop smoking, for example. If a medication is prescribed for you, take it, even if you don't feel any symptoms. If it is someone you love who has high blood pressure, your responsibility takes the form of being supportive of his or her efforts to change dietary and exercise habits and to follow any guidelines for medication.

Once you start a medication, your blood pressure will be monitored regularly so that you can be sure you are receiving the correct dosage. Sometimes medication, in combination with diet, exercise, and improvement in lifestyle, will reduce blood pressure enough so that the medication can be reduced or eliminated. Then you may be able to control your blood pressure with diet and exercise alone. Changing your lifestyle may be economical in the long run. If you *do not* treat the condition while it is still in an early stage, you may incur the costs of treating later complications.

WORKING TOWARD BETTER HEALTH

Now that you know you have high blood pressure you will

want to work closely with your doctor to bring it within a more normal range. Your doctor and health care team may have told you much of what is in this book. If you are like most of us, however, you don't absorb all of what you hear when you are excited or a little bewildered by a new disease. This book will reinforce what your doctor tells you. It may also answer some of the questions you forgot to ask and clarify some of the explanations you receive. In some instances information in this book may differ somewhat from what your doctor and health care team tell you, in which case you should discuss your concerns with them. They know you and your individual case best.

This book will help you work with your health care team for the best possible results—better health.

2

What Is Blood Pressure?

What is blood pressure, and why is normal blood pressure so important to your overall good health?

The term *blood pressure,* as used in medicine, refers to the force of your blood against the walls of your arteries, created by your heart as it pumps blood through your body. As your heart pumps or beats, the pressure increases. As your heart relaxes between beats the pressure decreases. High blood pressure, or hypertension, is the condition in which blood pressure rises too high and stays there.

YOUR PERSONAL ROAD MAP

Your circulatory system is a wondrous and intricate system responsible for the constant and appropriate distribution of approximately five quarts of blood throughout your body. Adequate flow of blood to every part of your body is necessary for optimum good health. This transportation system is composed of arteries, the largest channels that carry blood from the heart; narrower tubelike structures called *arterioles*; the microscopic capillaries; and finally the venules and larger veins, which carry blood back to the heart. You might visualize the network of vessels through which your blood flows from large arteries to capillaries as a tree with branches and twigs that get progressively smaller as they subdivide. The branches have greater diameters than the twigs, and finally tiny stemlike structures are connected to each leaf. Don't underestimate the importance of the tiny capillaries, because they bring oxygen and nutrients to the body cells and carry away waste products. If all the capillaries in your body were put together, they would be about 70,000 square feet or would form a ribbon a foot wide and 12 miles long.

WHAT IS BLOOD?

About half the volume of blood in the human body is made up of red and white corpuscles or cells. The remainder, called *plasma,* is a watery fluid surrounding the cells of the blood. Plasma contains many chemicals, hormones, and nutrients. Blood also contains cholesterol, a fatty substance that aids in the digestion of fats you eat, produces hormones, and prevents water from evaporating through your skin. Unfortunately, cholesterol, if excessive, may contribute to the formation of plaque on the inside walls of blood vessels, restricting blood circulation and contributing to hardening of the arteries and high blood pressure.

WHAT DOES BLOOD DO?

Your blood performs many functions, including gathering oxygen from your lungs and returning waste carbon dioxide to them. As your food is digested, blood carries the nutrients for use throughout your body. Waste products are then carried by your bloodstream and excreted from your body through the kidneys, intestines, skin, and lungs.

Signals for moving blood from various points and directing it to others are triggered by complex regulatory controls involving the nervous system and many hormones produced within your body. Blood helps you maintain the proper balance of chemicals and fluids, regulates body temperature, sends substances to fight infections when needed, and forms clots to stop loss of blood after injury.

YOUR HEART

Your heart is really not heart-shaped at all. It is about the size and shape of your fist in a clenched position and is located beneath your breastbone between your lungs. Your heart is a hollow, muscular organ that is quite different from other muscles in your body. Some of your muscles are voluntary, which means you can consciously control them. An example is the biceps muscle in your forearm. Other muscles are involuntary such as the muscles of your heart and around your blood vessels; you cannot control them. The unique muscle in your heart is known as the *myocardium*. This word was derived from two Greek words: *myo,* meaning muscle, and *cardio,* meaning heart.

Your heart muscle is arranged in thin sheets, one wrapped around the next, something like the layers of an onion. The fibers of one heart muscle sheet are perpendicular to the fibers of the sheet beneath. Because of this arrangement, the muscle of your heart contracts rhythmically about 100,000 times a day with a motion like that of a wet towel that is being wrung out. Blood is squeezed out of the heart chambers in a spiraling movement toward the openings of valves leading to your arteries. As your heart beats, its chambers alternately expand as they fill with blood and contract as blood is pumped out. With each beat blood leaving the heart is forced into large elastic arteries, which dilate in response to the rising pressure of the heart contraction, or *systole*. These arteries then contract elastically as the pressure falls during the period between beats, or *diastole*. The elastic stretching and recoiling of the arterial walls smooths out the flow of blood, allowing some flow during the diastolic interval, not only during the systolic.

Your heart has four chambers, and four valves control the flow of blood out of it and back into it again. The left and right sides each have an atrium, a chamber in which returning blood collects, and a ventricle, a chamber that pumps blood out. The right atrium receives venous blood from which body tissues have removed oxygen and added carbon dioxide. This blood then moves to the right ventricle, which pumps blood out of your heart and into the lungs, where carbon dioxide is eliminated and fresh oxygen is collected. Next, blood travels to the left atrium and into the left ventricle, from which it is pumped through the circulatory system to all parts of your body.

Your heart's pumping action is regulated by a small bundle of cells that generate electrical impulses. When your heart relaxes between beats the reduction of pressure causes blood to flow in. Valves permit blood from the right atrium to flow to the right ventricle and let blood from the left atrium flow to the left ventricle. Then the impulse to contract or squeeze reaches both atria, causing additional blood to move to the ventricles. Slightly later, as the ventricular muscle receives the signal to contract, valves between both atria and ventricles close. Blood is then forced out of the heart and toward the lungs from the right ventricle and to the rest of the body from the left ventricle.

When the normal flow of blood through the heart and, as a result, throughout the body is hindered in any way—for example, when the heart's beating mechanism is impaired or the blood supply to the heart is blocked—the condition is known as *cardiovascular disease*. Cardiovascular disease is dangerous because it may damage the brain, heart, kidneys, and other vital organs and tissues of the body.

YOUR ARTERIES

What you feel at your wrist as your pulse is actually the effect on your arteries produced by the pumping action of your heart. You can feel your pulse easily on the radial artery near your wrist by resting your left arm on a table with your palm up and placing the second and third fingers of your right hand over the artery.

The large arteries in your body have three layers, and it is the middle layer that is elastic enough to permit stretching to adjust to a larger volume of blood as soon as it is pumped from your heart. When your heart relaxes between beats these vessels narrow and force the blood to move forward.

Because of the elastic quality of your arteries, blood flow is continuous. Although variable, it doesn't start and stop. If the vessels were rigid like water pipes, blood would move mainly during the period of heart contraction, when the pumping action takes place.

The larger, more elastic arteries branch into smaller blood vessels, which are more muscular and less elastic. The intermediate-sized arteries are named for the organ to which they supply blood; for example, the renal artery goes to the kidneys, and the hepatic artery goes to the liver. As the arteries enter their target organ, they divide into small branches and eventually into even smaller vessels (the arterioles), which contain only a muscular layer and lining cells. Arterioles finally connect with the tiny microscopic capillaries composed only of lining cells. Tiny pores between these lining cells are large enough to permit passage of fluids, gases, and nutrients in and out of the bloodstream but small enough to prevent loss of red and white blood cells and plasma proteins that are carried in the blood. While arterioles are small, they are important because, by either constricting or relaxing their muscle cells, they can regulate their diameter and the flow of blood from the arteries into the capillaries, forcing the pressure in the arteries up or down. These arterioles and their tone, or degree of contraction or relaxation, are extremely important to the body in regulating the level of the pressure in the arterial system. Other body systems also greatly influence the blood pressure, as you will learn later in this book.

3

Measuring Blood Pressure

You don't feel your blood circulating through your body and usually do not feel symptoms of high blood pressure. The only effective way to measure your blood pressure is to have it checked with specially designed equipment.

HOW BLOOD PRESSURE IS MEASURED

Blood pressure is most often measured in the large artery in your upper arm with an instrument known as a *sphygmomanometer*. This piece of equipment consists of a squeeze-bulb pump, an inflatable cloth-covered rubber cuff, and a measuring device with a pressure gauge. The gauge measures millimeters of mercury (expressed as *mm Hg*). Some physicians use a sphygmomanometer in which the pressure is read from the height of an actual column of mercury. More common are sphygmomanometers employing a readout dial that has been calibrated against a mercury column standard.

The word *sphygmomanometer* was derived from two Greek words: *sphygmo,* referring to pulse, and *manometer,* referring to a measuring device. Measuring blood pressure isn't a new idea. The modern sphygmomanometer was invented in 1895. Other more primitive devices to estimate blood pressure existed before that.

To measure your blood pressure, the special cuff is wrapped around your upper arm and inflated with air until the flow of blood in your arm is temporarily stopped. As the air in the cuff is released gradually, an examiner listens with a stethoscope over the artery inside your elbow for the first sound of blood flowing through the artery. The number on the gauge at the first sound indicates the maximum pressure produced in the artery each time the blood is forced from the heart into the large blood vessels. This pumping pressure is known as the *systolic* pressure. More air is released slowly from the cuff. Within seconds all the pumping or beating sounds stop. At the time the sounds become inaudible the number on the pressure gauge indicates the resting or minimum blood pressure, known as *diastolic* pressure.

While both are important, your diastolic reading is more significant than the systolic, because the systolic level lasts only a short period, after which the pressure begins to fall rapidly toward the diastolic level. Your diastolic reading, taken when your heart is pausing, shows the lower but longer duration of pressure to which the heart and arteries are exposed. The higher the diastolic pressure, the higher the pressure against which the heart must work in order to eject blood into the general circulation. It is this increased heart effort and increased pressure within the arteries and arterioles that may ultimately cause accelerated and more severe atherosclerosis in the arterial system of the body and damage to the brain, kidneys, heart, and other vital organs.

HOW IS BLOOD PRESSURE EXPRESSED?

Standard blood pressure readings are expressed in figures representing the force required to raise a column of mercury (Hg) to a certain height, measured in millimeters (mm). Readings are expressed in numbers that look like a fraction but are not. The pumping pressure, or systolic pressure, is stated first, and the resting pressure, or diastolic pressure, is stated second. For example, your blood pressure may be 120/80. This would be expressed verbally as "one hundred twenty over eighty."

WHAT IS CONSIDERED NORMAL BLOOD PRESSURE?

Normal blood pressure varies from moment to moment within each individual. Your blood pressure may be higher at one time than another. It goes up when you exercise or are under stress and goes down when you rest or sleep. In an otherwise healthy adult, however, the generally recognized normal range of systolic (pumping) blood pressure is from 90 to 120 mm Hg; the diastolic (resting) blood pressure ranges from 55 to 90 mm Hg.

In determining whether you have high blood pressure, your physician will be concerned with the *usual* pressure in your system. Your physician may measure your blood pressure more than once during a visit. For example, if you have hurried to the office, you may feel out of breath, which could contribute to a high reading. Later during the visit, as you relax, your blood pressure may go down. Also, your physician may consider the average of several readings taken at different times before making a diagnosis of high blood pressure. If your blood pressure reading is high on only one occasion, your physician will want to measure your blood pressure again under other circumstances to see if drug treatment is necessary.

WHAT REGULATES BLOOD PRESSURE?

Your blood pressure varies throughout each day. When you are exercising and your body requires greater blood flow, the pressure increases. When you are resting, blood pressure decreases; it is lowest when you are asleep. It may change when you become excited, when you have a sudden injury, or after you smoke a cigarette. Many factors cause changes in the amount of blood your heart pumps as well as the state of the arterioles.

If you increase the amount of water flowing through a garden hose, you will increase the pressure in the hose. And if you decrease the diameter of the nozzle of the hose, you will increase the pressure in the rest of the hose. The quantity of blood being pumped and the diameter of your arteries are regulated by hormones secreted by various organs and glands and by your nervous system. Some hormones cause the diameter of your arterioles to decrease. They act on the thin layers of smooth muscle cells surrounding each arteriole, causing them to constrict, or squeeze together. Other nervous system and hormonal factors (parasympathetic nervous system and its hormones) cause arterioles to be less constricted and more dilated.

Your arteries and heart react to hormones and your nervous system and cause your blood pressure to go up or down. One hormone that causes squeezing of the smooth muscle cells of your arterioles is norepinephrine. You may recall reading about this hormone in psychology books. Together with epinephrine, this hormone is produced as a defense mechanism in what has been called the "fight or flight" reaction. When you are excited or more active more of it is secreted. As part of the body's alarm system this hormone goes directly to the arterioles to do its work.

YOUR HORMONES AND YOUR NERVOUS SYSTEM

Hormones also contribute to regulation of the amount of blood that your heart pumps. Norepinephrine is one of several hormones that affect blood pressure by varying the quantity of blood your heart pumps. Because your heart is composed mostly of muscle that is affected by hormones, hormones can cause it to contract more vigorously with each beat. More vigorous contractions mean that more blood is pumped with each beat.

Hormones also can change the total quantity of your blood. When the quantity increases, your heart pumps more blood and your blood pressure increases. Your kidney makes a hormone called *renin,* which increases blood volume because it causes your body to retain salt, which in turn causes retention of water. Some of this extra water joins your bloodstream and adds to the volume of blood in your body. Renin also causes formation of another hormone, angiotensin, which acts to constrict or squeeze the muscle cells of the arterioles.

Your arterioles and heart are also regulated by your nervous system, specifically your autonomic nervous system, over which you have no conscious control. In the presence of any type of stress, including excitement or exercise, your body increases the quantity of blood that is pumped by your heart, and blood pressure goes up. Your autonomic nervous system also is responsible for releasing the hormone norepinephrine, which causes veins to contract and blood to return to your heart more rapidly. This also increases the amount of blood pumped by your heart.

LOW BLOOD PRESSURE

Blood pressure that is *too* low can be just as dangerous as high blood pressure. How does low blood pressure occur? If your body loses blood, a drop in blood pressure may result because the blood volume is insufficient to fill the vascular space. Blood may be redistributed from parts of the body that still contain adequate supplies. The spleen, liver, and blood vessels of the gastrointestinal system may hold reserves of blood for such emergencies. After blood loss, fluids from the tissues are forced back into the blood vessels, helping to restore blood volume but reducing the concentration of red blood cells. This action may restore blood pressure to normal, but if the circulating volume of blood is insufficient to handle the demands of the entire body, the blood pressure may not be maintained, and a dangerous state of inadequate circulation, called *shock,* may develop.

When blood pressure is dangerously low a physician may prescribe a medication to constrict or squeeze blood vessels or may give red cells, whole blood, or fluids, depending on the cause of the lowered blood pressure.

Low blood pressure is only occasionally an extended medical problem, and much less frequent than is commonly assumed. Persons with a serious deficiency of adrenal cortex hormones or those with inadequate control of blood vessel tone in their legs are among the patients with chronic severe reduction of blood pressure resulting in disability. Many healthy persons have blood pressure in the lower normal range and have no symptoms or disability and no long-term predisposition to illness.

TYPES OF HIGH BLOOD PRESSURE

There are two types of hypertension, generally classified by cause. Hypertension may be known as *primary* or *secondary*. If you are an otherwise healthy person, your high blood pressure is known as primary hypertension. About 90 percent of all hypertensives are of this type, in whom the condition occurs for no obvious reason. While specific causes are unknown, primary hypertension *is* a disease, and it is important and possible to control it. Secondary hypertension is high blood pressure that is a symptom or an effect of a disease elsewhere in the body, such as in the kidneys.

HOW DOES HIGH BLOOD PRESSURE FEEL?

Because so many people don't feel any symptoms with high blood pressure, the disease has been called "the silent killer" by the American Heart Association. However, some people with advanced high blood pressure have persistent headaches, dizziness, fatigue, tension, and shortness of breath. These symptoms may also result from many other causes. The only way to know whether you have high blood pressure is to have your blood pressure checked.

CHECKUPS AND BLOOD PRESSURE TESTS

Although many people recognize that it is a good idea to have a checkup by a physician every several years, particularly after age 40, many do not do so. Many of us wait to schedule an appointment with our physician until we have a problem or a question. Many of us see a dentist more often than we see a doctor. We are aware of the need for good oral health and know what damage dental cavities and gingivitis (gum disease) can cause. However, the idea that hypertension is an undesirable condition seems more remote. In the early stages of high blood pressure we aren't motivated to see a physician because there is no pain or visible symptom.

The American Dental Association has encouraged its member dentists to take patients' blood pressure regularly. Dentists can have an important influence on patients. They have good relationships with their patients and can make necessary referrals to physicians. Many dentists have explained the problems associated with high blood pressure to their patients and have motivated many people experiencing the early stages of high blood pressure to seek medical attention.

In many communities local health departments have regular screening sessions to detect high blood pressure. *Screening* means measuring blood pressure for many individuals. Such programs usually refer persons identified as having high blood pressure to their physicians for further diagnosis and appropriate treatment. A high reading at such a screening on one occasion is a good indicator of potential trouble but does not necessarily mean that the person has high blood pressure. Perhaps you have been told about your blood pressure at such a screening program. If so, follow up with a visit to your physician. If your blood pressure reading is high on more than one occasion, your physician will probably want to do a further examination and may recommend dietary, exercise, and lifestyle changes as treatment. Medication may or may not be necessary. Each individual is different. What is effective for one person may be less effective for another. Treatment for high blood pressure is an individualized matter.

WHY YOU?

If you are among the 90 percent of individuals for whom the cause of high blood pressure isn't known, you may not get a satisfactory answer to the question "Why me?"

Are you overweight? Hypertension is more common in overweight people and in older people. However, thinner, younger people also suffer from hypertension. Did your parents or grandparents have high blood pressure? Sometimes it results from your genetic background. If your parents or siblings had it or have it, you are somewhat likelier to get it than those from other families.

Your sex and race also seem to make a difference. More men than women have high blood pressure, and more blacks than whites have it.

Are you diabetic? High blood pressure is more common in diabetics than among nondiabetics. Yet, while having diabetes alone isn't always enough to cause high blood pressure, in some cases diabetes can contribute directly to high blood pressure. If kidney disease is present, diabetics may also develop high blood pressure as a result of the loss of kidney function. Diabetics who use insulin injections or oral medication need not worry that these drugs cause or aggravate hypertension. Under a physician's supervision such interactions are carefully considered, thus preventing such side effects.

About 10 percent of cases of high blood pressure are related to another problem (secondary hypertension), such as inflammation or interference with blood flow through the kidney, a tumor of the adrenal gland, or a defect of the aorta. If the other problem can be corrected, blood pressure often returns to normal. If this cannot be accomplished, treatment to control the hypertension itself, as in primary hypertension, may be necessary.

The answer to the question "Why me?" depends on your heredity, your general state of health, and, to a large degree, your lifestyle. The components of your diet and the amount of exercise you get routinely may be important contributing factors in developing high blood pressure. Researchers have found that proper diet and adequate exercise play an important role not only in *treating* high blood pressure, but also in preventing it. Diet and exercise affect your arteries and arterioles, and it is the constriction of the arterioles that causes blood pressure to rise. If your blood pressure is high, your arterioles show more constriction than those in people whose blood pressure is within normal range.

Once you have been identified as having high blood pressure, it is important that you have it monitored regularly. Your physician will note the reading at the start of treatment and will refer back to past readings as time goes on to determine changes. How long does it take to reduce high blood pressure? How long did it take to get the way it is? With some adjustments in your eating, exercising, and smoking habits, and perhaps medication, changes will occur, possibly within a period as short as a few months. Depending on the severity of your case, it may take longer. How fast changes occur isn't as important as the fact that you are on the way to a healthier lifestyle.

4

Reduce Your Personal Risk Factors

The term *risk factor* may have come into use as a result of the study done in Framingham, Massachusetts, in which statistics showed that each of five health risk factors interacted with each other to increase the likelihood of heart attack. High blood pressure, cigarette smoking, excess body weight, high serum cholesterol level, and diabetes were identified as the risk factors. These risks are additive. This means that having any one factor increases your chances of heart attack, and the more factors, the greater the risk. Of all the risk factors, however, high blood pressure is considered the most significant.

While you are helping yourself to health by trying to bring your blood pressure under control you will also want to consider how you stand with regard to the risk factors. Do you smoke? If so, stop. Are you overweight? Then lose weight. Do you eat foods with a high fat content? Cut down on them. Do you have diabetes? Have you had your blood sugar level checked lately? If it is high, follow your physician's recommendations for bringing it under control. You *can* control the other major risk factors. There are many ways you can help yourself.

SMOKING: IT'S YOUR CHOICE

Smoking is a major threat to your health, probably a more important one than you think. The cigarette you smoke causes a chain of events throughout your body. The nicotine makes your heart beat faster, forcing your heart to work harder and require more oxygen. At the same time the carbon monoxide from the tobacco smoke reduces the amount of oxygen carried by your blood to your heart and other tissues. This situation is made even worse by the fact that smokers are more likely than nonsmokers to have hardening of the arteries, which are narrowed by a buildup of fatty deposits on their inner walls. Your heart then must work even harder to pump blood through narrowed blood vessels. This condition, atherosclerosis, is the major cause of heart attack and stroke, according to the American Heart Association.

Other major health organizations take a position on smoking and high blood pressure. For example, the High Blood Pressure Information Center of the National Institutes of Health has issued a direct statement regarding this effect: "Smoking injures your blood vessel walls and speeds up hardening of the arteries. The acute effect of a few cigarettes on blood pressure may be slight, but chain smoking significantly speeds the pulse rate, increases the work of the heart, and raises the blood pressure. People with hypertension just should not smoke."

When blood vessels are narrowed, blood cannot flow as effectively to the arm and leg muscles, causing a circulatory condition of the arms and legs known as *peripheral vascular disease.* Most people with this disease who develop some form of blockage in their arteries are smokers, says the American Heart Association.

People with diabetes who smoke cigarettes are at even greater risk for peripheral vascular disease. If you have hypertension *and* diabetes, your physician will outline a treatment plan to reduce your high blood pressure as well as your high glucose level, but to be sure the plan is effective you will want to stop smoking to reduce your combined risk factors.

Heart attack—those are two dramatic words. Are they enough to make you stop smoking? The American Heart Association says that cigarette smoking increases the risk of heart attack even more if you also have high blood pressure and/or high blood cholesterol. Your cholesterol level can be reduced through dietary means and perhaps medication. Your high blood pressure can be controlled, under your physician's supervision, with diet, exercise, and a few changes in your lifestyle. The cigarette habit is your choice.

When your heart muscles do not get enough oxygen because of narrowed heart arteries (coronary arteries), a condition called *angina pectoris* can occur. Chest pain is the characteristic signal of the condition. However, even before the pain occurs, cigarette smoking can reduce your level of physical capability because it reduces the amount of oxygen going to the heart muscle and makes the heart beat faster.

Chronic lung diseases, such as bronchitis and emphysema, interfere with oxygen transport and put additional pressures on the heart. These lung diseases are worsened by smoking. You can break this chain of events by not smoking.

Researchers advise women who use oral contraceptive pills not to smoke because the combination of using the pills and smoking cigarettes increases a woman's risk of heart attack even more.

The time to begin reducing the risk factor of smoking is during youth. To young people the risk of a heart attack usually seems remote. However, teenagers who smoke cigarettes begin to develop early signs of disease that can lead to later problems. As long as you continue to smoke, coughing, decreased stamina, and a fast heart rate build into chronic lung disease or heart disease.

The American Heart Association says that no cigarettes are safe, even the low-tar and low-nicotine cigarettes, because many smokers smoke more and inhale more deeply when they switch to these. Thus the smoker is exposed to more of the other harmful substances in the smoke that may increase risks of disease.

Why Quit Smoking Now?

Cigarette smoking gives you a two-to-six-times greater risk of heart attack than that faced by a nonsmoker. If you smoke more than a pack a day, you increase your risk of heart disease threefold. According to the American Cancer Society, cigarette smoking also increases your risk of *fatal* heart attacks over that of a nonsmoker. How long you smoked and the amount you smoked each day may play a role in your risk factor. If you never had a heart attack and you quit smoking now, your risk of a heart attack in the future immediately goes down.

Changing your smoking habit can affect your overall physical condition. Exercise will be easier once you quit, because your breathing capacity will begin to increase. In turn, you will be able to exercise more, to the point at which you can achieve a training effect and strengthen your cardiovascular system.

No one ever said it was easy to stop smoking. If it was so easy, would there be so many "stop smoking" programs operated by both profit and nonprofit organizations? If you want to quit, the first step is to make the decision. Talk to your physician about local support groups. Or have someone you care about help support you in your effort. Don't store cigarettes or carry them with you. Don't carry a lighter or matches. Instead of smoking, chew sugarless gum or eat low-calorie snacks. Change your attitude about mixing smoking with social activities.

Your decision to stop smoking can mean a drastic reduction in your combined risk factors.

OBESITY: THE UNNECESSARY WEIGHT

Obesity is considered a risk factor for developing heart disease because extra pounds make your heart work harder and less effectively. High blood pressure is more common in overweight people. Generally, as an overweight person gains more weight, blood pressure tends to rise. When the person loses weight, blood pressure often goes down. For some people losing weight brings high blood pressure under control. If your blood pressure is only slightly elevated and you are overweight, losing weight may be all that is necessary, and you may not need medication. For some people taking high blood pressure medication, dosages can be reduced after weight loss. Reducing the dosage of a medication is a goal to strive for because a smaller dose means a smaller chance of side effects from the drugs.

By itself, being moderately overweight may not be very dangerous. But combined with high blood pressure and high cholesterol levels and cigarette smoking, the risks compound. The dangers of obesity are even greater if you also have diabetes. Losing extra pounds may help you reduce your blood pressure. It may also reduce your blood cholesterol level and help you fight the possibility of developing diabetes or, if you already have diabetes, win the battle in controlling that disease, too.

Why Lose Weight Now?

Maintaining your best weight can make you feel better, because it will keep you healthier. Maintaining a good weight is especially important if you have a family history of high blood pressure, heart disease, or stroke.

How to lose weight and stay on an appropriate diet for fat, cholesterol, and calorie reduction will be outlined in Chapter 6. Right now, just consider the risks of those unnecessary extra pounds, along with the risks of your high blood pressure.

CHOLESTEROL: A POTENTIAL ENEMY

Most Americans have developed eating patterns that include frequent servings of meat, eggs, and dairy products, which contain lipids (fatlike substances) known as cholesterol. These substances can form deposits on the walls of your arteries, narrowing them and raising your blood pressure. Once you have high blood pressure, narrowing of your arteries is an additional risk factor. To prevent your arteries from becoming clogged, your physician will probably advise you to reduce the amount of fatty foods in your daily diet.

A diet lower in cholesterol is an easy diet to live with. You can choose more foods such as lean chicken, fish, fruits, and vegetables. You don't have to omit meat from your diet unless your physician specifically advises you to do so. Use the leaner cuts of lamb, veal, and beef. Trim off all the visible fat on steaks or roasts served to you. Better yet, if you do the cooking, trim off the fat before the meat is cooked. When you prepare a soup or stew with meat, let it stand overnight in the refrigerator. A layer of fat will congeal and rise to the top. You can remove the hardened fat before warming the dish for serving.

You'll find more helpful hints about low-cholesterol foods and diets in Chapter 6. For now, remember that cholesterol is an additional risk factor, along with your high blood pressure. Make the choice now to reduce that factor.

DIABETES: IF YOU HAVE IT, CONTROL IT

Diabetes is a risk factor that, added to the risk of high blood pressure, can threaten your health. If you have diabetes, the supervision of your physician will be important in controlling it and minimizing the additive risk effect.

Diabetes is a disease in which the body is unable to use certain foods properly. Normally the main food constituents—carbohydrates, proteins, and fats—are converted in the body into a simple sugar called *glucose*. The hormone *insulin,* produced by the pancreas, is needed to store glucose or use it for energy. When diabetes develops, the body cannot make enough insulin or fully use the insulin that is produced. As a result abnormally high levels of glucose build up in the blood and also in the urine. With poorly controlled diabetes, recurrent or continued high levels of blood glucose may result over a period of time in serious complications, including kidney failure, heart disease, stroke, and eye disease.

Diabetes can be controlled through a careful balance of diet, exercise, and sometimes insulin or an antidiabetic oral medication.

Diabetes interacts with the other risk factors. For example, obesity is the leading cause of diabetes in people over age 40. Obesity also figures into the causes of high blood pressure. Many people have diabetes and don't know it. Many people also don't know they have high blood pressure. Having regular checkups that include blood pressure and glucose level tests can provide for early detection and treatment of both conditions.

CONTROLLING YOUR PERSONAL RISK FACTORS

Think of the risk factors for heart disease as a card game. You may have been dealt some bad cards, but how you play them is your choice. There is something you can do about them. Controlling your high blood pressure and helping yourself to health can depend on how you play your cards of weight control; diet control, including reduction of fats (as well as sodium and calories, as you will learn in Chapter 6); and controlling diabetes, if you have it. Smoking is not something life gave you. That was a choice you made for yourself. If you chose to smoke, you can now choose *not* to smoke.

In addition to these major risk factors, of course, aspects of your lifestyle play a role in controlling your high blood pressure. How exercise and better methods of coping with stress can help you will be discussed in Chapter 7.

Take your personal risk factor inventory, counting your high blood pressure as the first risk. Decide now to take some positive actions to help yourself to health.

5

The High Cost of Complications

High blood pressure can be an inexpensive disease to treat. You don't need any special equipment, and you don't always need medication. It may require only that you pay careful attention to the food you eat, get a little extra exercise, and lose some weight. You may be advised to quit smoking, perhaps to consume less alcoholic and caffeinated beverages, and possibly to take a medication. All that can fit into your budget without any extra strain.

Health care can become expensive, however, when blood pressure is untreated and uncontrolled. Since blood pressure is a variable characteristic, the risks of other diseases occurring are related to the degree to which the blood pressure is abnormally high. The risks of other complications are proportional to the level of your blood pressure. How you control your blood pressure and reduce the risks of complications is up to you. You can do it by choosing to follow a healthier lifestyle; that's something you can't buy.

Generally, the most costly complications associated with blood pressure elevation fall into the categories of heart, brain, kidney, and eye diseases.

SAVE YOUR HEART

In Chapter 2 you read about the arteries in your body and how their elasticity contributes to a continuous flow of blood to your vital organs. One of the greatest threats to the health of your heart is the disease of the circulatory system known as atherosclerosis. This condition occurs when fatty deposits form in the lining of the arteries and prevent a smooth flow or block the flow of blood. Atherosclerosis is more prevalent among populations that eat large amounts of animal fat and less common among people whose diet is lower in animal fat. With this information researchers say that this disease can be prevented—or its progress slowed—by eating foods lower in fat. (You will learn more about low-cholesterol diets in Chapter 6.) While there is no known causal connection between atherosclerosis and high blood pressure, atherosclerosis is generally more severe in the presence of high blood pressure. The two often occur together and can be treated together. One of the greatest dangers of atherosclerosis occurs when it affects the coronary arteries of the heart, where a blockage can cause a heart attack.

People with high blood pressure are statistically more likely to have a heart attack or stroke than people whose blood pressure is within a normal range. However, even people whose blood pressure is normal develop various forms of cardiovascular disease, including heart attack and stroke. No one is immune.

Heart attack occurs when there is a sudden lack of oxygen-carrying blood in one of the arteries leading to the heart muscles. The lack of oxygen damages the heart muscles supplied by that artery. The disease originates in the blood vessels carrying the blood to the heart, not in the heart itself.

Lack of oxygenated blood flow to the heart can occur for several reasons. Physicians often use any one of several specific terms to name what we generally label *heart attack*. The terms *coronary thrombosis, coronary occlusion,* and *myocardial infarc-*

tion are descriptive. The first two mean the same thing and describe the blocking of blood flow to the heart by an obstruction. Coronary thrombosis or coronary occlusion is the most common type of heart attack, in which a blood clot (or thrombus) blocks the flow of blood through a coronary artery to the heart muscle. The occlusion almost always occurs in a coronary artery previously narrowed by atherosclerosis. Myocardial infarction describes the effect of that stoppage of flow to the heart: localized heart muscle injury. Myocardial infarction may be the most descriptive term to identify a heart attack because it describes what is actually injured or diseased.

A heart attack is the most severe form of coronary disease. The word *coronary* means *shaped like a crown* and refers to the blood vessels that surround the heart, providing the oxygen and nourishment to its muscles, which allow it to beat. *Coronary heart disease* is a more general term for any long- or short-term condition in which too little blood and oxygen are carried to the heart muscle and is usually caused by narrowing of the blood vessels due to atherosclerosis.

Uncontrolled high blood pressure, coupled with a buildup of serum cholesterol, can intensify the risks of developing any of the forms of coronary heart disease. One form is called *angina pectoris,* and it occurs when the muscle fibers of the heart temporarily get insufficient blood through narrowed coronary arteries but without permanent damage to the heart muscle. The main symptom, usually induced by exertion and lasting a period of minutes, is a sensation of pressure, squeezing, or tightness, starting in the center of the chest under the breastbone and often radiating to the left arm or throat area. Persons with this condition are usually advised to reduce their blood pressure, reduce the amount of animal fat in their diet in an effort to prevent further narrowing of their blood vessels, reduce their weight, eliminate smoking, and remain closely monitored by their physicians. Many people with angina pectoris must avoid sudden strenuous activity and restrict their level of exertion to avoid a heart attack. The angina pain is similar to that felt during a myocardial infarction (heart attack). However, pain during an infarction is of longer duration, is more intense, and is not promptly responsive to nitroglycerine.

Coronary insufficiency denotes more prolonged episodes of inadequate coronary blood flow without permanent myocardial damage but which may eventually lead to a heart attack.

Congestive heart failure, a possible result of several forms of heart disease, including coronary heart disease, means that the heart cannot pump enough blood to meet the body's needs so that blood and fluid tend to accumulate in lungs, liver, legs, and body cavities, which, if untreated, may result in impaired function and possibly permanent heart damage.

Cardiac arrest is the term used when the heart stops any coordinated pumping. Emergency measures are necessary to try to start the heart beating again.

SAVE YOUR BRAIN

Sometimes the word *stroke* is wrongly confused with the term *heart attack*. Stroke refers to a cerebrovascular (brain and blood vessel) accident. The brain needs a constant flow of blood. When this flow is interrupted because of blocking of arteries or veins or by bleeding from a blood vessel into brain tissue, mental or body functions controlled by that portion of the brain are affected immediately. Atherosclerosis contributes to, or may complicate, the cause of stroke. Stroke can also result from several other causes, but the primary causes are weakened or narrowed blood vessel walls developing within the brain, or resulting from obstructing clots carried to the brain from within the heart or large arteries of the head and neck.

Signs of stroke vary, depending on the degree of blockage in the blood vessel. Signs may range from impairment of speech to paralysis of parts of the body. Some stroke victims regain all of their faculties; others do not.

Care for stroke and heart disease can be expensive. It can take time from your work, require hospitalization, and reduce your productivity. While many forms of heart disease are treatable, the best cure known is prevention.

You can save your heart as well as your brain by following the routine your physician recommends to reduce your high blood pressure, including lifesaving changes in your lifestyle.

SAVE YOUR KIDNEYS

Experts consider uncontrolled high blood pressure one of the leading causes of damage to the kidneys and eventual kidney failure. The major function of your kidneys is to eliminate waste products from your body through the formation of urine. They help maintain a balance of acid and alkaline conditions and the proper levels of important elements and fluids within the body. The kidneys themselves are important in regulating blood pressure.

Your kidneys are each about four inches by two inches by one inch (larger or smaller, depending on your body build). They are located high on the rear wall of your abdominal cavity. During each 24-hour period about 150 gallons of blood pass through them. About 10 percent of that blood is selectively removed and reabsorbed by kidney cells, and finally about 3 percent, or about one to two quarts, is secreted as urine, which contains waste products that must be removed from the body.

This filtration process is accomplished through a series of more than a million minute tubes and filters that depend on a constant and smooth flow of blood. High blood pressure can damage these tiny filtration units where urine is formed. When the arteries leading to the kidneys become narrowed and thickened, the blood supply to the kidneys is reduced, in turn reducing the amount of fluid they can filter. An abnormal fluid retention pattern occurs because salt tends to be retained instead of excreted. And, because salt tends to attract water, the fluid retention increases the chances for heart damage.

In time, kidney function deteriorates, and various types of kidney problems may occur. One of the most serious is uremia, which results when the toxic waste products accumulate in the blood instead of being excreted in the urine. When the kidneys fail, potassium is also retained. When the potassium reaches a certain level in the blood it has a poisonous effect on the heart, which can lead to heart failure.

Some people with advanced kidney conditions must undergo a special kidney treatment program called *dialysis* or have a kidney transplant, both of which are very expensive procedures.

SAVE YOUR EYES

One of the reasons your physician peers into your eyes with an instrument called an *ophthalmoscope* each time you have a complete physical examination is to look carefully at the tiny blood vessels on the surface of the retina at the back of your eyes. Often the first sign of damage from high blood pressure is observed in this way. Your eyes are one of the few places your doctor can actually see inside you. By looking through the opening of your pupil your doctor can see your blood vessels and observe if any changes have taken place. If any narrowing of blood vessels or tiny hemorrhages are present, this is an important clue to what might be happening throughout your body.

The minute blood vessels in your eyes can function only as well as your entire circulatory system functions. Without proper and adequate blood circulation tiny vessels can become narrowed and cut off the supply of nourishing blood to areas of the retina, the layer of nerve cells that perceive light. Over a period of time visual disturbances—even blindness—can occur. And deterioration of the retina is often associated with atherosclerosis and diabetes.

You can help save your eyes by reducing your personal risk factors. You can reduce your high blood pressure and, if you have diabetes, keep that under control as well. A balance of appropriate diet, exercise, medication (if prescribed), and a good mental attitude toward life will help you avoid further, costly complications.

SAVE YOUR JOB AND YOUR FAMILY LIFE

Because heart, brain, kidney, and eye complications can become serious, they often entail lost time from work, hospitalization, and long periods of treatment and recuperation. You can avoid the expenses of these situations—and mental anguish to your family—by following your physician's instructions for treating your high blood pressure. Keep the costs of your own personal health care down by taking care of your high blood pressure as soon as you have been advised to begin a treatment program. Your high blood pressure won't just go away. You have to help yourself to health.

6

Diet in Controlling Hypertension

If you enjoy eating, the word *diet* may cause your blood pressure to skyrocket. You may find the idea of changing your eating habits unappealing. As your physician will point out, however, your eating habits are very important to your health, whether or not you have hypertension. Your eating habits are essential to your continued good health if any of the following characteristics apply to you:

- You *do* have hypertension.
- You have any of the other major risk factors of coronary artery disease—a cigarette habit, a high cholesterol level, excess weight, or diabetes.
- You are burdened by stress and tension.
- You exercise too little.
- You have a kidney problem.

WHERE DO YOUR NUTRIENTS COME FROM?

All the nutrients in your body come from the foods you eat,

which can be divided into five groups that work together to make up a well-balanced diet:

- Meat, poultry, fish, beans
- Vegetables and fruit
- Bread and cereal
- Milk products and cheese
- Fats, oils, sweets, alcohol

The first four groups supply your body with the amount of vitamins, minerals, protein, and other nutrients your body needs. The fifth group, fats, sweets, and alcohol, provides very few essential nutrients not available in the others and mainly provides excess calories. Limiting items in this group is generally believed to be advantageous. Yet, some medical experts say that moderate alcohol drinking (one to two ounces per day) lowers the risk of hypertension. Such moderate drinkers have also been found to have higher levels of high-density lipoproteins (HDLs) in their blood, and these HDLs may protect them against atherosclerosis.

The American Heart Association has developed recommendations for protecting your heart by cutting down on the amount of meats, eggs, and dairy products you eat. The chart on pages 38–39 provides guidelines for a healthy diet that includes some of all the basic nutrients. Your physician might advise you to follow a diet something like this or to modify it further to meet your specific needs.

Don't let the word *diet* scare you. To control hypertension you don't need a special diet but rather one that is planned and followed carefully—using the same foods other people eat—to give you the best possible nutrients without the harmful effects of certain foods and habits.

If you have hypertension or want to avoid it, several aspects of your diet are important: salt, cholesterol and fats, and your weight. Excessive salt—or, more specifically, sodium, which comprises 40 percent of pure salt—has been linked with high blood pressure. High intake of cholesterol and fats has been linked with atherosclerosis. Additionally, your weight and the amount of

1 MEAT POULTRY FISH DRIED BEANS and PEAS NUTS · EGGS

1 serving . . .

3-4 ounces of cooked meat or fish (not including bone or fat) or 3-4 ounces of a vegetable listed here

Use 2 or more servings (a total of 6-8 ounces) daily

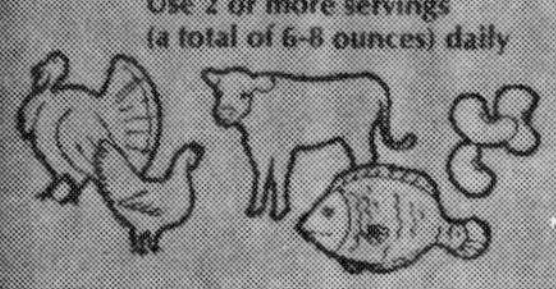

RECOMMENDED

Chicken • turkey • veal • fish • in most of your meat meals for the week.

Shellfish: clams • crab • lobster • oysters • scallops.

Use a 4-ounce serving as a substitute for meat.

Beef • lamb • pork • ham • less frequently.

Choose lean ground meat and lean cuts of meat • trim all visible fat before cooking • bake, broil, roast, or stew so that you can discard the fat which cooks out of the meat.

Nuts and dried beans and peas:

Kidney beans • lima beans • baked beans • lentils • chick peas (garbanzos) • split peas • are high in vegetable protein and may be used in place of meat occasionally.

Egg whites as desired.

AVOID OR USE SPARINGLY

Duck • goose

Shrimp is moderately high in cholesterol. Use a 4-ounce serving in a meat meal no more than once a week.

Heavily marbled and fatty meats • spare ribs • mutton • frankfurters • sausages • fatty hamburgers • bacon • luncheon meats.

Organ meats: liver • kidney • heart • sweetbreads • are very high in cholesterol. Since liver is very rich in vitamins and iron, it should not be eliminated from the diet completely. Use a 4-ounce serving in a meat meal no more than once a week.

Egg yolks: limit to 3 per week including eggs used in cooking.

Cakes, batters, sauces, and other foods containing egg yolks.

2 VEGETABLES and FRUIT

(Fresh, frozen, or canned)

1 serving . . . ½ cup

Use at least 4 servings daily

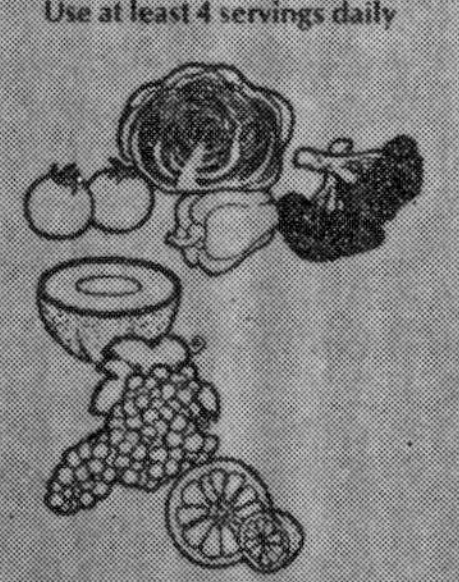

RECOMMENDED

One serving should be a source of Vitamin C:
Broccoli • cabbage (raw) • tomatoes. Berries • cantaloupe • grapefruit (or juice) • mango • melon • orange (or juice) • papaya • strawberries • tangerines.

One serving should be a source of Vitamin A—dark green leafy or yellow vegetables, or yellow fruits:
Broccoli • carrots • chard • chicory • escarole • greens (beet, collard, dandelion, mustard, turnip) • kale • peas • rutabagas • spinach • string beans • sweet potatoes and yams • watercress • winter squash • yellow corn.
Apricots • cantaloupe • mango • papaya.

Other vegetables and fruits are also very nutritious; they should be eaten in salads, main dishes, snacks, and desserts, *in addition* to the recommended daily allowances of high vitamin A and C vegetables and fruits.

AVOID OR USE SPARINGLY

If you must limit your calories, use vegetables such as potatoes, corn, or lima beans sparingly. To add variety to your diet, one serving (½ cup) of any one of these may be substituted for one serving of bread or cereals.

3 BREAD and CEREALS

(Whole grain, enriched, or restored)

1 serving of bread . . . 1 slice
1 serving of cereal . . .
½ cup, cooked
1 cup, cold,
with skimmed milk

Use at least 4 servings daily

RECOMMENDED

Breads made with a minimum of saturated fat:
White enriched (including raisin bread) • whole wheat • English muffins • French bread • Italian bread • oatmeal bread • pumpernickel • rye bread.

Biscuits, muffins, and griddle cakes made at home, using an allowed liquid oil as shortening.

Cereal (hot and cold) • rice • melba toast • matzo • pretzels.

Pasta: macaroni • noodles (except egg noodles) • spaghetti.

AVOID OR USE SPARINGLY

Butter rolls • commercial biscuits, muffins, donuts, sweet rolls, cakes, crackers • egg bread, cheese bread • commercial mixes containing dried eggs and whole milk.

*Reproduced with permission from the American Heart Association.

4 MILK PRODUCTS

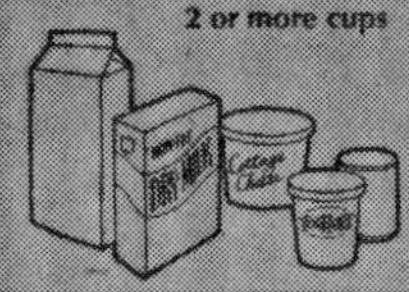

1 serving . . . 8 ounces (1 cup)

Buy only skimmed milk that has been fortified with Vitamins A and D.

Daily servings:
Children up to 12 . . .
    3 or more cups
Teenagers . . .
    4 or more cups
Adults . . .
    2 or more cups

RECOMMENDED

Milk products that are low in dairy fats:

Fortified skimmed (non-fat) milk and fortified skimmed milk powder • low-fat milk. The label on the container should show that the milk is fortified with Vitamins A and D. The word "fortified" alone is not enough.

Buttermilk made from skimmed milk • yogurt made from skimmed milk • canned evaporated skimmed milk • cocoa made with low-fat milk.

Cheeses made from skimmed or partially skimmed milk, such as cottage cheese, creamed or uncreamed (uncreamed, preferably) • farmer's, baker's, or hoop cheese • mozarella and sapsago cheeses. Processed modified fat cheeses (skimmed milk and polyunsaturated fat)

AVOID OR USE SPARINGLY

Whole milk and whole milk products:

Chocolate milk • canned whole milk • ice cream • all creams including sour, half and half, whipped • whole milk yogurt.

Non-dairy cream substitutes (usually contain coconut oil which is very high in saturated fat).

Cheeses made from cream or whole milk.

Butter.

---

5 FATS and OILS

(Polyunsaturated)

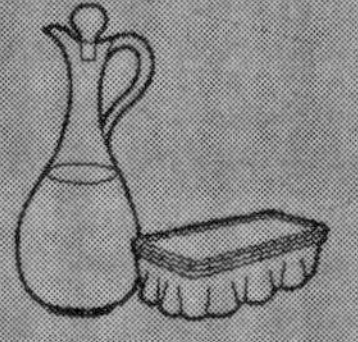

An individual allowance should include about 2-4 tablespoons daily (depending on how many calories you can afford) in the form of margarine, salad dressing, and shortening.

RECOMMENDED

Margarines, liquid oil shortenings, salad dressings and mayonnaise containing any of these polyunsaturated vegetable oils:

Corn oil • cottonseed oil • safflower oil • sesame seed oil • soybean oil • sunflower seed oil.

Margarines and other products high in polyunsaturates can usually be identified by their label which lists a recommended *liquid* vegetable oil as the *first* ingredient, and one or more partially hydrogenated vegetable oils as additional ingredients.

Diet margarines are low in calories because they are low in fat. Therefore it takes twice as much diet margarine to supply the polyunsaturates contained in a recommended margarine.

AVOID OR USE SPARINGLY

Solid fats and shortenings:

Butter • lard • salt pork fat • meat fat • completely hydrogenated margarines and vegetable shortenings • products containing coconut oil.

Peanut oil and olive oil may be used occasionally for flavor, but they are low in polyunsaturates and do not take the place of the recommended oils.

---

6 DESSERTS BEVERAGES SNACKS CONDIMENTS

The foods on this list are acceptable because they are low in saturated fat and cholesterol. If you have eaten your daily allowance from the first five lists, however these foods will be in excess of your nutritional needs, and many of them also may exceed your calorie limits for maintaining a desirable weight. If you must limit your calories, limit your portions of the foods on this list as well.

Moderation should be observed especially in the use of alcoholic drinks, ice milk, sherbet, sweets, and bottled drinks.

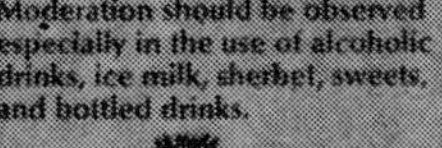

ACCEPTABLE

Low in calories or no calories

Fresh fruit and fruit canned without sugar • tea, coffee (no cream), cocoa powder • water ices • gelatin • fruit whip • puddings made with non-fat milk • low calorie drinks • • vinegar, mustard, ketchup, herbs, spices.

High in calories

Frozen or canned fruit with sugar added • jelly, jam, marmalade, honey • pure sugar candy such as gum drops, hard candy, mint patties (not chocolate) • imitation ice cream made with safflower oil • cakes, pies, cookies, and puddings made with polyunsaturated fat in place of solid shortening • angel food cake • nuts, especially walnuts • peanut butter • bottled drinks • fruit drinks • ice milk • sherbet • wine, beer, whiskey.

AVOID OR USE SPARINGLY

Coconut and coconut oil • commercial cakes, pies, cookies, and mixes • frozen cream pies • commercially fried foods such as potato chips and other deep fried snacks • whole milk puddings • chocolate pudding (high in cocoa butter and therefore high in saturated fat) • ice cream.

calories you consume may contribute to coronary artery disease as well as to hypertension.

SHAKE YOUR FINGER AT THE SHAKER

Your doctor may have advised you to cut down on sodium-rich foods as part of your diet to control your blood pressure. Doing so may be easier than you think. Most of us in the United States eat much more salt than we need. However, because numerous studies have linked a high salt or sodium diet with hypertension, more Americans are shaking their fingers at the shaker.

What is salt? A molecule of salt is simply one atom of chlorine attached to one atom of sodium. The two atoms separate when they dissolve in the blood or other body fluids. Since the sodium atom makes up only four-tenths of the molecule's weight, pure salt is 40 percent sodium.

Salt (sodium) is important to your body's proper functioning. For example, it is largely responsible for retaining water in your body. By attracting water into the blood vessels, the element helps to maintain blood volume and pressure.

You need only about 200 milligrams of sodium per day, yet most adults in the United States consume 4,000–8,000 mg of sodium per day (more than 16 pounds of salt a year). The American Medical Association considers less than 4,800 mg of sodium per day as the level of moderation for the healthy adult. To give you an idea of how much sodium that is, 1 teaspoon of salt contains 2,130 mg of sodium.

You were not born with your taste for salt; you acquired it. Cow's milk has more salt than breast milk, so most of us acquire the taste for salt very early in life. According to some researchers, too much salt at an early age can aggravate a predisposition toward (or susceptibility to) hypertension. Inbred hypertension-prone laboratory rats fed high-salt diets soon developed high blood pressure. Other studies indicate that eating too much salt early in life can set a bad pattern for later life. In response to this issue baby food manufacturers recently reduced the amount of salt in baby foods.

In many of the more primitive societies in remote areas of the world, sodium intake is low. For example, the Kalahari Bushmen of South Africa, the Melanesian tribes of New Guinea, and Eskimos in Alaska consume between 200–1,400 mg of sodium per day. In these societies, hypertension is almost unheard of. In northern Japan, however, where the daily intake of sodium averages over 9,000 mg, there is about twice the incidence of hypertension as in the United States. Studies have shown that when primitive societies adopt more modern ways of life, including an increased sodium intake, blood pressure increases.

Only in the last several thousand years has modern man salted his food. At times salt was scarce and therefore valuable. The Romans used salt instead of money to pay their soldiers. The word *salary* was derived from the Latin word for salt, *salarium*.

Over the centuries salt has become important and, as the Salt Institute points out, it is the oldest known food additive. Salt is said to bring out the natural flavor in many foods. Salt is also an important preservative that checks microorganisms that could spoil or poison many foods. Salt helps to develop the color, especially in processed meats, that we have come to expect. In sausage salt acts as a binder. In many foods it aids texture. It also regulates fermentation in the processing of foods such as pickles, sauerkraut, sausage, cheese, and bread dough. With the addition of sodium some chemicals and drugs are made more stable— chemicals such as sodium saccharin (a sweetener), sodium bicarbonate (an antacid), MSG (monosodium glutamate, a flavor enhancer), and sodium pentobarbitol (a sedative).

Especially high in sodium content are prepackaged and processed foods. Canned and fast foods top the list. For example, one cup of canned tomato sauce has almost 1,500 mg of salt. Eating out can increase your salt intake unexpectedly. For example, a chicken dinner at a fast food restaurant can contain more than 2,200 mg of sodium—10 times the sodium you need in a single day.

Animals in the wild get very little sodium, especially those animals that eat plants, vegetables, and fruits, which are very low in sodium (an apple contains only 2 mg of sodium; an ear of corn, also 2 mg; 10 grapes, 1 mg). Yet the food we buy for our pets has added salt in it.

Some athletes occasionally take salt tablets to replace salt lost through perspiration during strenuous exercise. However, according to researchers, the quantity of electrolytes (salt is an electrolyte) lost through sweating is more than adequately resupplied by the food we eat. In addition, athletes who take too much extra salt risk dehydrating themselves further.

We are often unknowingly exposed to an excess of sodium. For example, according to researchers at Texas A & M, 40 percent of the U.S. population's tap water may contain more sodium than we need. Water softeners contribute additional sodium, but this can be avoided by a special tap that bypasses the water softener.

Sodium and Calorie Content of Common Foods

Food Item	Common Measure (Weight, g)	Sodium, mg	Calories
Beverages (Alcoholic)			
Beer, regular	12-oz can or bottle (360)	18	151†
Beer, light	12-oz can or bottle (360)	14	70-136†
Brandy	1½ fl oz (45)	1	105
Gin (86 proof)	1½ fl oz (45)	1	105
Rum (86 proof)	1½ fl oz (45)	1	105
Vodka (86 proof)	1½ fl oz (45)	Trace	105
Whiskey, bourbon, rye, or scotch (86 proof)	1½ fl oz (45)	1	105
Wine, red domestic	4 fl oz (120)	12	99
Wine, red imported	4 fl oz (120)	6	99
Wine, sherry	4 fl oz (120)	14	161
Wine, white domestic	4 fl oz (120)	19	99
Wine, white imported	4 fl oz (120)	2	99
Beverages (Nonalcoholic)			
Apple juice	6 fl oz (180)	4	87
Coffee, brewed	1 cup—8 fl oz (240)	2	0
Coffee, instant	1 cup—8 fl oz (240)	1	2
Cranberry juice cocktail	6 fl oz (180)	3	123
Grape juice, bottled or canned	6 fl oz (190)	6	125
Orange juice, fresh	6 fl oz (180)	4	84
Orange juice, frozen	6 fl oz (186)	4	92
Pineapple juice	6 fl oz (188)	3	69
Prune juice	6 fl oz (192)	4	149
Soft drink‡			
Regular	8 fl oz (240)	11	96
Diet	8 fl oz (240)	29	1
Club soda	8 fl oz (240)	56	0
Collins mix	8 fl oz (240)	20	112
Quinine water (tonic)	8 fl oz (240)	2	72
Mineral water	8 fl oz (240)	42	0
Tomato juice	6 fl oz (192)	659	36
Tea	1 cup—8 fl oz (240)	1	0
Tea, instant	1 cup—8 fl oz (240)	2	0
Vegetable juice cocktail	6 fl oz (182)	665	30

Sodium and Calorie Content of Common Foods (continued)

Food Item	Common Measure (Weight, g)	Sodium, mg	Calories
Breads and Crackers			
Biscuit, home recipe	1 biscuit (28)	175	103
Biscuit, mix, with milk	1 biscuit (28)	272	104
Bread, French	1 slice (23)	116	64
Bread, pumpernickel	1 slice (32)	182	79
Bread, rye	1 slice (25)	139	61
Bread, white	1 slice (25)	114	76
Bread, whole wheat	1 slice (25)	132	61
Bread stick, salt coating	1 stick, small (10)	167	38
Bread stick, without salt coating	1 stick, small (10)	70	38
Cracker, saltine or soda	1 cracker (3)	35	12
Cracker, soup or oyster	10 crackers (8)	83	33
Roll, dinner, brown and serve	1 roll (28)	138	83
Roll, frankfurter, hamburger	1 roll (40)	202	119
Roll, hard	1 roll (50)	313	156
Cereals (Non-Sugar-Coated)§			
Bran, all	1 oz—⅓ cup (28)	160	70
Bran flakes (40%)	1 oz—⅔ cup (28)	265	90
Corn flakes	1 oz—1 cup (28)	350	110
Corn Chex	1 oz—1 cup (28)	325	110
Granola	1 oz—¼ cup (28)	75	130
Grits, cooked	1 oz—¾ cup (28)	10	100
Oat flakes	1 oz—⅔ cup (28)	275	100
Oatmeal, regular, without salt	1 oz—⅓ cup (28)	1	109
Oatmeal, instant, regular flavor (salt added)	1 oz—¾ cup (28)	252	105
Rice, cream of, unsalted	1 oz—¾ cup (28)	10	110
Rice, puffed	½ oz—1 heaping cup (14)	10	50
Rice Chex	1 oz—1⅛ cup (28)	275	110
Rice Crispies	1 oz—1 cup (28)	340	110
Wheat Chex	1 oz—⅔ cup (28)	240	110
Wheat, cream of, regular	1 oz—¾ cup (28)	7	110
Wheat flakes	1 oz—1 cup (28)	370	110
Wheat, puffed	½ oz—1 heaping cup (14)	10	50
Wheat, shredded	1 large biscuit (21)	1	80
Condiments, Dressings, and Seasonings			
Barbeque sauce	1 tbsp (16)	130	14
Catsup, tomato	1 tbsp (15)	156	16
Chili sauce	1 tbsp (17)	227	16
Mayonnaise	1 tbsp (15)	78	101
Mustard, prepared	1 tsp (5)	65	5
Parsley flakes	1 tbsp (4)	2	2
Pepper, black	1 tsp (2)	1	8
Salad dressings			
Bleu cheese or Roquefort	1 tbsp (15)	153	76
French	1 tbsp (14)	214	66
Italian	1 tbsp (15)	116	83
Russian	1 tbsp (15)	133	74

Sodium and Calorie Content of Common Foods (continued)

Food Item	Common Measure (Weight, g)	Sodium, mg	Calories
Thousand Island	1 tbsp (16)	109	80
Oil and vinegar	1 tbsp (15)	Trace	62
Salt, table	1 tsp (6)	2,325	0
Soy sauce	1 tbsp (18)	1,029	12
Sugar, granulated	1 tsp (4)	Trace	15
Worcestershire sauce	1 tbsp (17)	206	Trace
Dairy Products, Eggs,‖ and Margarine¶			
Butter, regular	1 tbsp (14)	116	102
Butter, whipped	1 tbsp (9)	74	69
Butter, unsalted, regular	1 tbsp (14)	2	102
Cheese, American	1 slice—1 oz (28)	406	116
Cheese, cheddar	1 oz (28)	176	114
Cheese, cottage	½ cup (113)	457	117
Cheese, cream	1 oz (28)	84	99
Cheese, parmesan, grated	1 oz (28)	528	129
Cheese, Swiss	1 oz (28)	74	107
Cheese, processed spread	1 oz (28)	381	82
Cream, half and half	1 tbsp (15)	7	20
Cream, heavy	1 tbsp (15)	6	53
Cream, sour	1 tbsp (12)	6	26
Egg, whole	1 medium (50)	69	79
Egg, white	1 medium (33)	50	16
Egg, yolk	1 medium (17)	8	63
Margarine, regular	1 tbsp (14)	133	100
Margarine, soft, tub	1 tbsp (14)	152	100
Margarine, unsalted	1 tbsp (14)	1	100
Milk, buttermilk	8 fl oz (245)	257	99
Milk, low-fat (2%)	8 fl oz (244)	122	121
Milk, skim	8 fl oz (245)	126	86
Milk, whole	8 fl oz (244)	120	150
Desserts#			
Brownies	1 average (20)	50	97
Cake, angel food	1 slice, ¹⁄₁₂ cake (56)	134	150
Cake, devil's food, chocolate icing	1 slice, ¹⁄₁₂ cake (67)	120	260
Cake, pound	1 medium slice (55)	171	225
Cake, white, white icing	1 slice, ¹⁄₁₂ cake (104)	243	290
Cake, yellow, with caramel icing	1 slice, ¹⁄₁₂ cake (108)	79	391
Cookies, chocolate chip	1 cookie, medium (11)	35	50
Cookies, sandwich	1 cookie (10)	40	63
Cookies, oatmeal	1 cookie (13)	27	120
Cookies, sugar	1 cookie (26)	108	128
Cookies, fig	1 bar (14)	48	56
Cookies, vanilla wafer	1 wafer (4)	9	16
Cookies, shortbread	1 cookie (8)	29	37
Gelatin, plain	½ cup (120)	60**	80
Ice cream	1 cup (140)	112	257
Ice milk	1 cup (131)	105	199

Sodium and Calorie Content of Common Foods (continued)

Food Item	Common Measure (Weight, g)	Sodium, mg	Calories
Pie, apple	1 slice, ⅛ pie (71)	208	182
Pie, banana cream	1 slice, ⅙ pie (66)	90	128
Pie, blueberry	1 slice, ⅛ pie (71)	163	172
Pie, cherry	1 slice, ⅛ pie (71)	169	185
Pie, chocolate cream	1 slice, ⅙ pie (66)	80	174
Pie, lemon meringue	1 slice, ⅛ pie (105)	296	268
Pie, mince	1 slice, ⅛ pie (71)	241	259
Pie, peach	1 slice, ⅛ pie (71)	169	150
Pie, pecan	1 slice, ⅛ pie (71)	241	259
Pie, pumpkin	1 slice, ⅛ pie (71)	169	150
Pudding, bread	½ cup (133)	267	248
Pudding, chocolate, home recipe	½ cup (130)	73	198
Pudding, chocolate, mix	½ cup (148)	195	322
Pudding, rice	½ cup (132)	94	194
Pudding, tapioca	½ cup (83)	129	111
Pudding, vanilla, home recipe	½ cup (128)	83	142
Pudding, vanilla, mix	½ cup (148)	200	321
Sherbet, orange	1 cup (193)	89	259
Fish and Seafood			
Bluefish, broiled or baked with butter	4 oz (114)	117	219
Clams, raw	4 to 5—3 oz (85)	174	56
Cod, broiled with butter	4 oz (114)	125	99
Crabmeat, canned, drained	1 can—4 oz (114)	1,250	126
Flounder, baked with butter	4 oz (114)	268	102
Haddock, fried	4 oz (114)	200	162
Halibut, broiled with butter	4 oz (114)	152	191
Lobster, boiled, meat only	4 oz (114)	183	123
Oysters, fresh	6 small—2 oz (58)	75	38
Salmon, broiled or baked with butter	4 oz (114)	133	207
Sardines, drained	1 can—3¼ oz (92)	598	187
Scallops, bay, steamed	10 to 12—4 oz (114)	302	153
Shrimp, raw	10 jumbo—3 oz (85)	137	98
Tuna, chunk, canned in oil, drained	1 can—3¼ oz (92)	328	182
Tuna, chunk, canned in water, drained	1 can—3¼ oz (92)	312	117
Fruits			
Apple	1 medium (138)	2	118
Applesauce, sweetened	½ cup (125)	3	227
Apricots, canned, syrup	½ cup (129)	13	111
Apricots, dried	5 halves, medium (24)	2	62
Banana	1 medium (119)	2	68
Blackberries	½ cup (72)	1	42
Blueberries	½ cup (72)	1	45
Cantaloupe	½ melon (272)	24	47

Sodium and Calorie Content of Common Foods (continued)

Food Item	Common Measure (Weight, g)	Sodium, mg	Calories
Cherries, sweet, whole	1 cup (130)	2	82
Cherries, canned	1 cup (257)	10	110
Fruit cocktail, canned in syrup	1 cup (255)	15	195
Fruit cocktail, canned in water	1 cup (255)	15	95
Grapefruit	½ grapefruit (120)	1	26
Grapefruit, canned	½ cup (127)	2	89
Grapes	10 grapes (50)	1	23
Honeydew	⅕ melon (298)	28	61
Orange	1 medium (131)	1	47
Peach, skinned	1 medium (100)	1	29
Peaches, canned, syrup	½ cup (128)	8	100
Peaches, canned, water	½ cup (128)	8	38
Pear	1 medium (168)	1	93
Pears, canned, syrup	½ cup (128)	8	98
Pears, canned, water	½ cup (128)	8	40
Pineapple, fresh	1 cup (135)	1	71
Pineapple, canned, syrup	1 cup (255)	4	189
Pineapple, canned, water	1 cup (246)	4	96
Plums	10 plums (66)	1	30
Plums, canned, water	1 cup (256)	10	111
Prunes, cooked	½ cup (107)	4	108
Prunes, dried	5 prunes (43)	2	95
Raisins	¼ cup, packed (36)	4	98
Rhubarb, cooked, sweetened	½ cup (135)	3	190
Strawberries	½ cup (75)	1	28
Strawberries, frozen, sweetened	½ cup (128)	1	139
Watermelon	¹⁄₁₆ melon (426)	8	55
Meat and Poultry			
Bacon, regular	2 slices—½ oz (14)	274	61
Bacon, Canadian	1 slice—1 oz (28)	394	58
Bologna	1 slice (22)	224	61
Beef, corned	2 slices—3 oz (85)	802	315
Beef, fried, creamed	1 cup (245)	1,754	377
Beef, ground, lean	1 patty—4 oz (114)	76	249
Beef, lean, rump roast	2 slices—4 oz (114)	74	237
Beef, lean, round steak	6 oz (170)	180	444
Chicken, broiler	¼ chicken (147)	58	120
Chicken, roasted	½ breast (98)	69	99
Chicken, fried	1 drumstick (56)	49	88
Frankfurter, all meat	1 frankfurter (57)	639	176
Ham, cured lean	2 slices—4 oz (114)	1,494	330
Ham, cured, country, lean	2 slices—4 oz (144)	980	304
Ham, fresh, lean	2 slices—4 oz (114)	79	426
Ham, chopped, lunchmeat	1 slice (21)	288	62
Ham, deviled	1 oz (28)	253	100
Lamb, loin chop, lean	2 chops—4 oz (114)	79	214
Lamb, leg, lean	2 slices—4 oz (114)	78	212
Liver, calf, fried	3 slices—4 oz (114)	133	298
Liver, chicken, simmered	5 livers—4 oz (114)	56	188

Sodium and Calorie Content of Common Foods (continued)

Food Item	Common Measure (Weight, g)	Sodium, mg	Calories
Liverwurst (braunschweiger)	1 slice (28)	324	88
Pork, loin roast, lean	1 slice—4 oz (114)	93	292
Salami, dry, beef and pork	1 slice (10)	226	45
Salami, cooked, beef and pork	1 slice (22)	255	88
Sausage, pork	1 link (13)	168	65
Sausage, pork	1 patty—2 oz (57)	259	129
Thuringer (summer sausage)	1 slice (22)	320	68
Turkey, dark meat	3 slices—4 oz (114)	91	218
Turkey, light meat	3 slices—4 oz (114)	61	200
Turkey, roll	1 oz (28)	166	70
Veal, cutlet, loin	1 cutlet—4 oz (114)	93	267
Pasta			
Macaroni, plain, cooked	1 cup (140)	2	155
Macaroni with cheese	1 cup (200)	1,086	430
Pizza with cheese	1 slice—2 oz (57)	380	147
Pizza with sausage	1 slice—2 oz (57)	335	157
Spaghetti, with tomato sauce and cheese	1 cup (250)	955	190
Spaghetti, with tomato sauce, meatballs, and cheese	1 cup (248)	1,009	332
Soups, Commercial Varieties, Condensed **(Prepared With Addition of Equal Volumes of Water, Unless Noted)**			
Bean	1 cup (250)	1,008	168
Beef broth	1 cup (241)	1,152	64
Chicken, cream of (with milk)	1 cup (245)	1,054	179
Chicken noodle	1 cup (240)	1,107	62
Chicken with rice	1 cup (241)	814	48
Clam chowder, Manhattan	1 cup (244)	938	81
Clam chowder, New England (with milk)	1 cup (248)	992	139
Minestrone	1 cup (241)	911	105
Mushroom, cream of (with milk)	1 cup (248)	992	216
Onion	1 cup (240)	1,051	65
Pea, green	1 cup (250)	987	130
Tomato	1 cup (245)	872	88
Tomato, cream of (with milk)	1 cup (250)	932	173
Turkey noodle	1 cup (240)	998	79
Vegetable beef	1 cup (245)	957	78
Vegetarian vegetable	1 cup (245)	823	78
Vegetables (Considered Fresh, Unless Listed Otherwise; Considered Cooked, Unless Indicated as Raw. Sodium Content of Cooked Vegetables is Content Before Salt is Added.)			
Artichoke	1 bud (120)	36	12
Asparagus	4 spears (60)	4	12
Asparagus, canned	4 spears (80)	298	17
Beans, baked, canned, with pork and tomato sauce	½ cup (145)	464	156
Beans, baked, canned, with pork and molasses sauce	½ cup (145)	303	192

Sodium and Calorie Content of Common Foods (continued)

Food Item	Common Measure (Weight, g)	Sodium, mg	Calories
Beans, green	½ cup (63)	3	16
Beans, green, canned	½ cup (65)	319	16
Beans, green, frozen	½ cup (68)	1	17
Beans, lima	½ cup (85)	1	95
Beans, lima, canned	½ cup (85)	228	82
Beans, lima, frozen	½ cup (85)	64	84
Beets	½ cup (85)	37	27
Beets, canned	½ cup (85)	240	42
Broccoli	1 stalk, medium (151)	18	39
Broccoli, frozen	½ cup (94)	18	24
Brussels sprouts	4 sprouts (84)	8	30
Brussels sprouts, frozen	½ cup (77)	8	26
Cabbage	½ cup (72)	8	16
Cabbage, raw	½ cup (35)	4	11
Carrots	½ cup (78)	26	34
Carrots, frozen	½ cup (113)	52	35
Carrots, raw	1 medium (72)	34	12
Cauliflower	½ cup (63)	6	14
Cauliflower, frozen	½ cup (90)	9	16
Cauliflower, raw	½ cup (58)	8	14
Celery, raw	1 stalk (20)	25	7
Corn	1 ear (140)	1	70
Corn, canned, creamed	½ cup (128)	336	105
Corn, canned, whole kernel	½ cup (83)	192	87
Cucumber, raw	6 large slices (28)	2	4
Lettuce, head, raw	¼ head (135)	12	18
Lettuce, leaf, raw	1 cup (55)	5	10
Mushrooms	½ cup (35)	4	10
Okra	5 pods (53)	1	16
Onions, green, raw, with tops	2 medium (30)	2	14
Onions, raw	1 tbsp (10)	1	4
Peas, green	½ cup (80)	1	57
Peas, green, canned	½ cup (85)	247	82
Peas, green, frozen	½ cup (85)	106	55
Peppers, sweet	½ cup (75)	13	22
Pickles, dill	1 spear (30)	232	3
Pickles, sweet gherkin	1 whole pickle (15)	128	22
Potato, baked or boiled	1 medium (156)	5	145
Potatoes, french fried, unsalted	10 strips (50)	15	137
Potatoes, mashed, milk and salt added	1 cup (210)	632	137
Radishes, raw	5 medium (18)	8	7
Sauerkraut	½ cup (235)	777	21
Spinach, canned	½ cup (103)	455	25
Spinach, frozen	½ cup (50)	78	24
Spinach, raw	½ cup (55)	25	7
Squash, summer	½ cup (105)	3	13
Sweet potato, boiled	1 medium (132)	20	126
Sweet potato, canned	1 medium (100)	48	107

Sodium and Calorie Content of Common Foods (continued)

Food Item	Common Measure (Weight, g)	Sodium, mg	Calories
Tomato, raw	1 medium (123)	14	27
Tomatoes, canned	½ cup (120)	195	26
Snacks			
Caramels, plain or chocolate	1 oz (28)	74	113
Candy, milk chocolate	1 oz (28)	28	147
Corn chips, regular	1 oz (28)	231	157
Doughnuts, cake type, plain	1 doughnut (32)	160	125
Mints, chocolate-coated	1 small (11)	20	45
Nuts, cashews, dry-roasted, salted	4 tbsp—1 oz (28)	150	159
Peanut butter	1 tbsp—1 oz (16)	81	94
Peanuts, dry-roasted, salted	4 tbsp—1 oz (28)	123	166
Peanuts, roasted in oil, unsalted	4 tbsp—1 oz (28)	1	208
Popcorn, salted with butter	1 cup (9)	175	41
Popcorn, unsalted	1 cup (6)	1	23
Potato chips	14 chips—1 oz (28)	285	161
Pretzels, regular twist	5 pretzels—½ oz (14)	505	117

Source: The Salt Institute, from data calculated by the U.S. Department of Agriculture.

*Values calculated from US Department of Agriculture Home and Garden Bulletin 233, *The Sodium Content of Foods,* 1980, and USDA Agriculture Handbook No. 456, 1975, unless otherwise noted.

†Values do not include sodium contributed by the base water, which varies according to geographic location.

‡Values, provided by the National Soft Drink Association, are average and do not include sodium contributed by the base water, which varies according to geographic location.

§Data provided by cereal companies.

‖From USDA Agriculture Handbook 8-1, *Composition of Foods, Dairy Products and Egg Products, Raw, Processed, Prepared,* revised 1976.

¶From USDA Agriculture Handbook 8-4, *Composition of Foods, Fats and Oils, Raw, Processed, Prepared,* revised 1976.

#Cake and cookie values from USDA Handbook 8-1, revised 1976.

**Sodium value varies with different fruit flavorings.

Lick the Salt and Sodium Habit

To help bring your blood pressure under control you'll want to lick the salt habit. Remember that most processed foods contain more sodium than nonprocessed foods. Fresh, frozen, and canned fruits and fruit juices are low in sodium. Most fresh and frozen vegetables are relatively low in sodium, but canned vegetables or frozen vegetables with a sauce are higher (140–460 mg per ½-cup serving). Grains are naturally low in sodium, though ready-to-eat and instant or quick cereals are generally higher in sodium (100–360 mg per ½-cup serving). Bread contains moderate levels of sodium. Most natural cheese is moderate to high in sodium content (75–300 mg an ounce), but processed cheeses and creamed and low-fat cottage cheese are much higher (350–450 mg an ounce).

Sausages, luncheon meats, frankfurters, and other cured meats such as ham contain larger amounts of sodium than fresh meats because salt is generally added as a preservative during processing. A 3-ounce serving may have as much as 1,350 mg of sodium.

Convenience foods and fast foods routinely contain more sodium than the other foods you eat.

Condiments can harbor huge amounts of sodium. For example, soy sauce contains more than 1,000 mg of sodium per tablespoon. Steak sauce, mustard, catsup, tartar sauce, and most other sauces have 125–250 mg of sodium per tablespoon. If you use condiments freely, consider how quickly this can add up. If you choose a salad because vegetables and fruits are low in sodium, hold the salad dressing. Most salad dressings have the same amount of sodium (125–250 mg per tablespoon) as other sauces.

In addition to the sodium already contained in foods, some estimates suggest that as much as one-third of the average daily intake of sodium comes from salt *added* to food in cooking or at the table. Many of us habitually upend our salt shakers over just about everything we eat. Many of us do this in the kitchen as well as at the table, often without even tasting before salting. As an alternative, learn to use spices and herbs or lemon juice instead of salt when seasoning. Seasoning with herbs, spices, or lemon juice may be preferable to using a salt substitute. Many cooks say salt substitutes, while adding a salty taste, also tend to impart a bitter taste to the food.

Many supermarkets today carry special low-sodium or salt-free foods. However, because these foods are specialty items, you may find them more expensive. The best way may be to eat more natural foods, such as fresh fruits and vegetables, and control the seasoning yourself.

For persons with high blood pressure on a <u>low salt</u> diet
you <u>may</u> have:*

1. Fresh Vegetables:
asparagus, barley, broccoli, carrots, cabbage, corn, cucumber, cauliflower, eggplant, green beans, green pepper, lettuce, mushrooms, navy beans, onions, peas, potatoes, parsley, spinach, squash, tomatoes, turnip greens, zucchini, frozen vegetables without salt.

2. Fresh Fruit:
apples, apricots, bananas, blackberries, blueberries, cherries, cantaloupe, cranberries, lemons, grapefruit, grapes, oranges, raspberries, peaches, pears, pineapple, watermelon.

3. Meats:
chicken, beef, lamb, duck, veal, quail, turkey, liver.

4. Fresh Fish

5. Cereal Products:
bread made without salt or with sodium-free baking powder, unsalted grits, oatmeal, puffed rice, puffed wheat, shredded wheat, rice, unsalted crackers, farina, macaroni, spaghetti.

6. Dairy Products:
non-fat dry milk, skim milk, evaporated milk, unsalted margarine.

7. Beverages:
coffee, tea, lemonade.

8. Spices:
garlic, pepper, onion powder, and all spices that do <u>not</u> contain <u>salt</u>.

For persons with high blood pressure on a <u>low salt</u> diet
you <u>may not</u> have:*

1. Table Salt

2. Meats:
salted or smoked meats, bacon or bacon fat, ham, salt pork, sausages, <u>all</u> luncheon meats, chipped and corned beef, frankfurters.

3. Fish that is salted or smoked.

4. Snack Foods:
potato chips or sticks, pretzels, salted nuts, salted popcorn, corn chips, crackers.

5. Relishes or Condiments:
pickles, olives, ketchup, soy sauce, worcestershire sauce, chili sauce, prepared mustard, sauerkraut, maraschino cherries, meat tenderizers.

6. Dairy Foods:
all cheeses, whole milk, ice cream.

7. Spices with "Salt":
celery salt, garlic salt, onion salt.

8. Cereal Products:
all commercial cereals or breads that contain salt, self-rising flour.

9. Alka Seltzer

10. Miscellaneous:
baking soda, baking powder.

6. Dairy Foods:
all cheeses, whole milk, ice cream.

7. Spices with "Salt":
celery salt, garlic salt, onion salt.

8. Cereal Products:
all commercial cereals or breads that contain salt, self-rising flour.

9. Alka Seltzer

10. Miscellaneous:
baking soda, baking powder.

*Source: Department of Hypertension and Nephrology, The Cleveland Clinic, Cleveland, Ohio.

Foods to eat (high in potassium and low in sodium)*

Fruits and Fruit Juices

Apples
Apricots
**Avocados
**Bananas
**Cantaloupe
Dates
Grapefruit
**Honeydew melon

**Nectarines
Prunes
**Raisins
Watermelon
Apple juice
**Grapefruit juice
Prune juice
Orange juice

Vegetables

Asparagus
Beans (white or green)
Broccoli
Brussel sprouts
Cabbage (cooked)
Cauliflower (cooked
Corn on the cob

Eggplant (cooked)
Lima beans (fresh and cooked)
Peas (green, fresh, and cooked)
Peppers
**Potatoes (baked or broiled)
Radishes
Squash (summer and winter, cooked)

Foods to avoid (high in potassium but also high in sodium or salt)*

Tomato juice, canned
Clams (raw)
Sardines
Lima beans (frozen)
Peas (frozen)
Spinach (canned)
Carrots (canned)

*Source: Department of Hypertension and Nephrology, The Cleveland Clinic, Cleveland, Ohio.
**Especially helpful

Dining Away from Home*

It is possible for you to remain on your sodium restricted diet, even though you may eat some of your meals in a restaurant. Your ability to choose foods wisely will increase as you become more familiar with your diet. Here are a few helpful hints:

1. Avoid obvious foods high in sodium; for example, olives, pickles, tomato juice, soup, crackers, potato chips, ham, and sausage.

2. *Do not* add table salt. Take your own salt substitute along with you.

3. Choose foods lower in sodium; for example:
    Fruit salads
    Raw vegetables
    Tossed salad with vinegar and oil dressing
    Baked potato
    Milk, tea, coffee (caffeinated or decaffeinated)
    Broiled steak or chop without seasonings
    Inside slice of roast beef, fresh pork, or roast chicken or turkey
        (no gravy)

4. Ask if it is possible that your food be prepared without added salt or sodium seasonings.

5. When you know you will be eating out, adjust the sodium content of foods eaten at home, choosing foods lower in sodium.

6. If you are allowed one-quarter teaspoon salt to use at the table, omit this allowance on the days you will eat out. This will help compensate for salt added while food is cooked.

7. Chinese food is usually high in sodium content, so avoid it if possible.

Spices can be added instead of salt to add flavor to your food. Most cookbooks give ideas of compatible seasonings for specific foods. Try them! You will be surprised at how much fun they can be. Here are some examples:

Beef:	Bay leaf, thyme, marjoram, onion, dry mustard, parsley, or dill
Pork:	Garlic, marjoram, or sage
Poultry:	Fresh or dried celery leaves, basil, marjoram, parsley, rosemary, summer savory, sage, thyme, or paprika
Fish:	Lemon, garlic, chopped dill, basil, or tarragon leaves
Tomatoes:	Garlic, onion, parsley, basil, sage, chervil, or tarragon
Carrots:	Chives, parsley, mint, or chervil
Corn:	Chives, parsley, green pepper, onion, tomato, or chili powder
Green beans:	Dill, thyme, marjoram, nutmeg, onion, chives, scallions, rosemary, lemon, or unsalted French dressing
Potatoes:	Parsley, chives, onion, rosemary, mace, or scallions

* Source: Department of Hypertension and Nephrology, The Cleveland Clinic, Cleveland, Ohio.

When cutting down on the salt you use in cooking, don't do it suddenly. Instead, cut it gradually. Just as you learned to like salt, you can also unlearn it. It may take a month or two, but you will gradually appreciate the difference. Many people contend that salt actually masks the fine taste of many foods. Therefore, once you have licked your taste for salt, you may actually enjoy the taste of your food more. Some researchers believe the taste buds may actually become more sensitive with less salt in the diet.

CHOLESTEROL AND FATS: FRIEND AND FOE

If your physician has advised you to reduce your cholesterol and fat intake, doing so will help you bring your blood pressure under control.

Cholesterol is a well-known fatlike substance. Cholesterol has many functions. It is necessary to the manufacture of essential hormones, it is an integral part of cellular membranes, and it is part of the fatty sheath that surrounds and insulates nerve cells. If you do not obtain enough cholesterol in the food you eat, your body manufactures it.

However, cholesterol is beneficial only up to a point. A high level of cholesterol in your blood and blood vessels is one of the risk factors of atherosclerosis and coronary artery disease. In atherosclerosis fats flowing in the blood may be deposited in the walls of the blood vessels. The vessels narrow, stiffen, and scar, and blood can no longer get through adequately. This resistance drives your blood pressure up. If you continue to consume foods high in fats and cholesterol, higher blood pressure aggravates and intensifies atherosclerosis and artery disease.

Experts have studied the populations of more industrialized countries, such as the United States, where people eat many foods rich in cholesterol. Here there are higher levels of blood cholesterol and higher rates of heart attacks than in less advanced countries, where people consume fewer calories and fewer animal products and have lower blood cholesterol levels and lower rates of heart disease.

Try to Eat Less Fat

Diets that contain lower levels of fats are linked with lower levels of blood cholesterol and are possibly linked with less risk of heart disease.

The two types of fat you hear about most often are saturated fats and polyunsaturated fats. Saturated fats, which are usually solid at room temperature, are mostly of animal origin, such as butter and fat on meat. Cholesterol occurs mainly in foods of animal origin. Polyunsaturated fats usually come from vegetable sources, such as vegetable oils. Until recently, researchers said that saturated fats were bad and polyunsaturated fats were good for you. Now, however, the issue is less clear, though most doctors generally recommend that their patients cut down on saturated fats.

Your doctor will tell you about the importance of eating less fat, reducing your sodium, and eating foods containing less sugar. A combination of these habits can contribute to a diet that will enable you to lose weight, another important aspect of controlling high blood pressure.

DIABETES: A MAJOR RISK FACTOR

Hypertension occurs more frequently in diabetics than in non-diabetics. If you are obese, your likelihood of being diabetic is greater than if you are thin. If you have diabetes (a disease in which your body cannot properly handle sugar), you have a major risk factor for hypertension and other heart problems. Diabetes increases your risk of heart attack and stroke and may lead to high blood fat levels, which, in turn, may lead to atherosclerosis and hypertension.

If you have diabetes, you can control it under your doctor's supervision by maintaining a low blood cholesterol level and a low-calorie intake.

OBESITY MAKES YOUR HEART WORK HARDER

If you are overweight, your doctor may ask you to lose weight as one of the first steps in treating your high blood pressure. Losing weight isn't enough. As the Heart, Lung, and Blood Institute of the National Institutes of Health points out, while lowering weight sometimes brings high blood pressure under control, it will not *control* it permanently. If you gain the weight back, you will also regain the high blood pressure.

Obesity places an added burden on your heart because your blood volume increases with your body weight, and your body's fat reserves must be supplied with blood. Consequently, the heart of an overweight person is forced to pump more blood through a much larger system of blood vessels. Blood pressure often rises as weight goes up.

CUTTING DOWN ON SUGAR

Are you one of the Americans consuming an average of more than 125 pounds of sugar a year? From 1960 to 1977 annual per capita consumption of caloric sweeteners in the United States increased by 22 pounds, mostly as a result of sweeteners added to commercially prepared foods and increased consumption of foods such as soft drinks.

How can you cut down on the amount of sugar in your diet? Watch labels. Sugar hides. Sugar is not the only word to look for. Watch for words such as *sucrose, glucose, fructose, dextrose, corn syrups, corn sweeteners, natural sweeteners,* and *invert sugar.* Some foods containing a lot of sugar may not taste sweet. Examples are catsup, salad dressings, and some peanut butters.

Go easy on pies, cakes, pastries, and cookies and try to avoid fruits canned in heavy syrup. As an alternative, try fruits canned in their own juice or other fruit juices. Limit your consumption of candy, jams, jellies, syrups, sweet toppings, soft drinks, and other highly sugared beverages.

Many cereals are presweetened. Check labels. Buy the unsweetened kind so *you* can control the amount of sugar added.

LOSING WEIGHT: MODERATION AND COMMON SENSE ARE THE KEY

Once you have decided to alter your diet you may want assistance in planning to lose weight, in shopping, and in cooking.

Probably the most important thing to remember is the principle of moderation. You put those pounds on slowly; that's how you should take them off. Beware of fad or miracle diets. While they may seem to work at first, they usually don't work over a long period of time. Some diets may be so dramatic that they are hazardous.

Losing weight simply means taking in fewer calories than you require to maintain your weight. You might say that 3,500 calories equals about one pound. If you use up 3,500 calories more than you need over a period of time you will lose one pound. What you choose to omit from your diet is an individual choice. (See Chapter 8 for how exercise and calories relate.)

When you go grocery shopping, prepare a list and follow it. On the shelves of your supermarket more than 10,000 food products beckon as a result of millions of dollars invested in market research and advertising. The odds are probably against your better judgment, especially if you are hungry when you shop.

When you have a meal, eat slowly. If there is still food on your plate when you're finished, save it. Ask for a doggie bag if you are in a restaurant.

While eating together is a pleasant social interaction, try to separate eating from social activities. Meeting a friend for a piece of pie with a cup of coffee is a sure way to add excess calories.

Become acquainted with a calorie chart. You need not become a calorie-watching fanatic, but your ability to judge caloric contents of foods will improve.

Finally, remember that the earlier you start forming a good habit, the more likely you are to continue it. If you have children, encourage them to form healthy eating habits. Obese children often become obese adults. A child with high blood pressure is likely to have high blood pressure as an adult, unless it is checked at an early age. Weight control may be one of the easiest—and least costly—ways to ensure future good health.

COOKBOOKS AND OTHER RESOURCES

Probably the best way to become aware of the salt, sugar, fat, and calorie levels in the food you eat is to do most of your own shopping and cooking. When you select and prepare your food you are not only more aware of the nutritional values of your food; you also control what goes into what you eat.

If you want information on cooking, there are good cookbooks and diet books that can assist you in controlling your weight and your sodium intake and thus hypertension. By following guidelines in the books you can also help others in your family avoid hypertension (see Chapter 9).

7

Control Your High Blood Pressure through Exercise and Lifestyle Changes

Just as your diet can affect your blood pressure and related risk factors, so too can your lifestyle, which includes the exercise you do, the stresses you face, and how you cope with those stresses. You'll want to make exercise a part of your life while you help yourself to health and reduce your high blood pressure.

EXERCISE AND HIGH BLOOD PRESSURE

Exercise is important because it improves the condition of your heart muscle and blood circulation and aids in utilizing calories and fats. Losing weight enables your heart to work more efficiently. Exercise and weight loss together can contribute to a reduction in blood pressure.

Champion athletes often have systolic blood pressures of 100 or lower. Similarly, hypertensive patients who exercise moderately can experience significant blood pressure reductions.

Exercise burns up calories. For example, if you walk briskly for a minute, you can burn up five or six calories. Coupled with the proper diet, exercise can help you maintain your present weight or lose some of it. Don't be concerned that the additional exercise will increase your appetite and thus your weight. Many people tend to desire less food once they are in better physical shape.

Exercise offers other benefits to your body as well. For example, exercise also appears to increase the level of high-density lipoproteins (HDLs) in your blood and reduce the levels of low-density lipoproteins (LDLs). Runners and joggers often have a higher blood level of HDLs than inactive people. A lipoprotein is made up of a lipid (*lipo*), or fat, molecule and a protein molecule. Fat molecules are not soluble in water; they bind to these lipoproteins, and that is how they are carried through the blood. There are two major types of lipoproteins. Low-density lipoproteins (the LDLs) are the proteins that carry most of the cholesterol throughout your body. Higher levels of these LDLs may promote atherosclerosis, perhaps because they do not do a very good job of carrying cholesterol. High-density lipoproteins (HDLs) are believed to reduce the risk of atherosclerosis, perhaps because they are more efficient at carrying cholesterol.

Many scientists believe that frequent exercise will help you develop collateral blood vessels in your coronary circulatory system. With more vessels supplying your heart muscle you are much more likely to survive if one of the coronary arteries supplying blood to your heart becomes blocked.

Exercise also strengthens your heart muscle. Sudden death associated with running for a bus or shoveling snow may not necessarily be the result of an actual blockage of a major blood vessel. It may come from a sudden, abnormally rapid heart rhythm resulting in insufficient coronary circulation in a heart that is not accustomed to being stressed. A well-conditioned heart is much less likely to go into these sudden rhythm changes, but there are exceptions.

Like any other muscle, the heart can become more efficient after exercise, or training. It will learn to do the same amount of work with less effort or expenditure of oxygen. Your overall endurance and stamina will increase, and your heart will be able to work longer and harder, with less fatigue. It will pump more powerfully, and your heart rate will go down. Pulses of long-distance runners may be as low as 30–40 beats per minute, while the average sedentary person's pulse may be 60–70 beats per minute.

Human history backs up the necessity for most of us to exercise. We started out as hunters. We chased, caught, and killed our food. All this involved a great deal of physical activity. Later we evolved into agricultural societies. Long hours and strenuous work were required in farming. Today mechanization and automation have set in. Many of us do little or no physical work. Typing, picking up telephones, filing, and sitting through long meetings is not the kind of exercise our ancestors had. Therefore it is necessary to add exercise to our daily lives.

Getting Started

If you are over age 40, your doctor may recommend an exercise stress test before you begin any new strenuous activities. Many doctors recommend them for middle-aged sedentary patients before they embark on an exercise program. A stress test consists of carefully graded running on a treadmill or pedaling a stationary bicycle. During and after this test an electrocardiogram (EKG) is taken. As you are running or pedaling your doctor will note your maximum heart rate.

If you don't take the stress test, there is a simpler way of estimating your maximum heart rate. Subtract your age from the number 220. For instance, if you are a 40-year-old man, your maximum heart rate should be about 180 beats per minute.

To reach the level of training effect at which your body and cardiovascular system are actually strengthened you should consider several things. First the exercise should be aerobic, or exercise that uses oxygen to help create energy for your muscles. This type of exercise increases the efficiency of your heart, muscles, lungs, and blood vessels. You must not exceed the level at which you are constantly supplying your muscles with sufficient oxygen to continue working. The exercise should be dynamic (as opposed to so-called isometric exercise such as weightlifting) and rhythmic. Your muscles should be used repeatedly. Sports that involve many muscles are preferable. Running, fast walking, cycling, swimming, and paced calisthenics are examples of aerobic exercise. You must exercise for 20–30 minutes at least three times a week, and the level of exercise should be such that your heart beats at 70–80 percent of its maximum rate. Take the example of the 40-year-old man again. His theoretical maximum heart rate is 180. The 70–80 percent range for that would be 126–153 beats per minute. While you're exercising, your heart rate should be within that range—70–85 percent of maximum. You can use your middle finger to read the pulse from your wrist or neck. Count the beats in 10 seconds and multiply by 6 to get your pulse per minute. If you have questions about this, discuss them with your health care team. They can also tell you what ideal heart rate you should try to achieve when exercising.

What is good exercise?

When you think of exercise you may have visions of all those people you see running each morning and evening. Running doesn't have to be your form of exercise. If running doesn't appeal to you, join a gym. You might like to use the athletic equipment. You might enjoy a team sport, such as volleyball or softball, or a racquet sport, such as tennis, racquetball, or squash. Swimming is also an excellent overall exercise and can be enjoyed throughout the year with the use of indoor pools in most areas. You might consider joining a health club, gym, or community center with athletic facilities.

Don't overlook the value of walking. There are those who "speedwalk" as fast as some can run. You can develop a walking routine. Take a walk early in the morning or late in the evening each day. Walk short distances instead of getting into your car. Walk the stairs instead of taking elevators. Try to do more exercise instead of less. With cars and elevators so available, many of us tend to forget that some distances are short and are manageable with foot power.

Most important, enjoy the exercise you choose. Discuss your likes and dislikes with your physician and health care team. They will help you adapt your interests to a program that will meet your needs and enable you to have fun at the same time.

Start Slowly

If you are interested in simple exercise to get into better shape and lose weight but are not interested in attaining a significant training effect, there are still some prerequisites to consider. Begin your exercise program with a warm-up by stretching and loosening up your various muscle groups. Exercise slowly at first. Before you are ready to stop, cool down slowly, allowing any muscles that are overworked and tense from exhaustion to relax. Exercise regularly, at least three times per week.

Taking Off Pounds

In Chapter 6 you learned that for every 3,500 calories burned you may lose one pound. With the table on page 64, you can determine how various exercises can help you utilize calories. Remember, however, that the calories used per hour are only an approximation and do not take into account your age, sex, body build, and how strenuously you participate in the activities stated.

Hints about Healthful Exercise

While exercise is generally beneficial, there are times when it can be harmful. For example, it can be dangerous to exercise in the heat in a sweat suit that increases heat and sweating. While you do sweat profusely, you lose water weight, which you will regain when you satiate your thirst later. Also, if you lose too much water in working out and sweating, such a loss, if not replaced promptly, can lead to dehydration, heat exhaustion, or heat stroke in extreme situations.

Good exercise habits, like good diet habits, should begin as early as possible in life. If you are a parent, encourage good exercise habits, because they lead to good health.

How Exercise Burns Calories

Activities		Calories Expended Per Hour
Strolling 1 mph Light housework	Walking 2 mph	120–150
Typing, manual Riding lawn mower	Golf, using power cart	150–240
Cleaning windows Mopping floors Vacuuming Pushing light power mower Bowling	Walking 3 mph Cycling 6 mph Golf, pulling cart Horseback (sitting to trot)	240–300
Scrubbing floors Walking 3.5 mph Cycling 8 mph Table tennis Badminton	Golf, carrying clubs Tennis, doubles Calisthenics (many) Ballet exercises Volleyball	300–360
Walking 4 mph Cycling 10 mph Ice skating	Roller skating Horseback ("posting" to trot)	360–420
Hand lawn-mowing Walking 5 mph Cycling 11 mph	Tennis, singles Water skiing	420–480
Sawing hardwood Jogging 5 mph Cycling 12 mph Downhill skiing	Paddleball Horseback (gallop) Basketball Mountain climbing	480–600
Running 5.5 mph	Cycling 13 mph	600–660
Running 6 or more mph Handball	Squash Ski touring (5 + mph)	Above 660

Select exercises that you enjoy; don't torture yourself with exercises that seem like hard work. If you choose an exercise that you can do alone but find you're quitting too easily or becoming bored with it, do it with a family member or friend.

STRESS AND TENSION

People with hypertension do not always have a high degree of tension or stress in their lives. That the word *tension* appears in the word *hypertension* is a coincidence that often misleads people. Even the most relaxed person can have hypertension. However, researchers have long suspected that stress and tension may influence blood pressure and lead to coronary artery disease and heart attacks.

A stressful situation may cause your blood pressure to rise. In most people blood pressure returns to normal after the stress subsides. If stress becomes a way of life for you, however, it is an additional risk factor for developing high blood pressure.

What is stressful for one person may not be for another, whether it is making a speech, having a job interview, or coping with a difficult job situation. Some of us do not cope with stress, fear, or anxiety very well; some of us have a more vulnerable temperament than others. Many of us become accustomed to responding to daily life as if it were a series of emergencies.

Some of us really do experience constant stress. An example is the air traffic controllers, whose jobs are notoriously stressful. A study was done at Boston University Medical Center in which the controllers freely carried on their work while researchers watched the controllers' pulse and blood pressure. The result: the controllers' incidence of high blood pressure was four times that of the average individual.

Stress is also known to raise blood cholesterol levels, which in turn contribute to heart disease. Studies involving blood analyses have shown increased blood cholesterol among medical students during critical examinations. Keep calm, keep cool, and keep your serum cholesterol down.

Controlling Stress and Hypertension

Arterial blood vessels carrying blood away from your heart are surrounded by muscle fibers. When the muscle fibers are relaxed the arterial vessels are slightly dilated and can carry a larger volume of blood. When the muscle fibers contract the arterial vessels shrink in diameter and resist blood flow, which in turn increases blood pressure. The tone of these blood vessels is controlled automatically by your autonomic nervous system, the system that also helps to control your heart.

Special nerve cells known as *baroreceptors* (*baro* = pressure) located in your blood vessels also help to regulate your blood pressure. They can detect changes in your blood pressure. Just as the thermostat in your home keeps the temperature from varying too much, baroreceptors constantly relay information to your autonomic nervous system, which controls the muscle fibers along your arterial blood vessels.

The objective of the baroreceptors is to keep your blood pressure within the narrow range they read as "normal." If your blood pressure suddenly goes up, they act through your autonomic nervous system to dilate blood vessels and slow your heart. If your blood pressure suddenly drops, as in shock, the baroreceptors rapidly notify the autonomic nervous system to speed up your heart rate and constrict your arterial vessels, pulling your blood pressure back up.

If you are continually under stress and your blood pressure rises repeatedly, your baroreceptors may reset themselves at a higher level and regard elevated blood pressure as normal. Once reset they may sustain new, higher blood pressure. According to the National Institutes of Health, there is growing evidence that these baroreceptors become less sensitive when they are constantly exposed to high blood pressure, allowing higher levels than they would have before.

Hormones may also influence your blood pressure. At times of strenuous exercise and high stress, such as fright, norepinephrine, epinephrine, and aldosterone are released into your blood in increased quantities. Aldosterone signals your body to retain water and sodium; the other two hormones are very powerful heart stimulants and blood vessel constrictors.

When these various regulatory systems go out of balance, hypertension can result.

Personality Type and Hypertension

Your personality may determine whether or not you develop hypertension and heart disease. About 20 years ago Meyer Friedman and Ray H. Rosenman, two California cardiologists, defined Type A and Type B persons. Type A persons, they said, suffered from two to three times as much heart disease as Type B persons. Type A persons don't handle stress as well as Type B persons. Over the years Friedman and Rosenman's hypothesis has been strengthened by other studies and evidence. Results of one such recent study found that Type A men have more atherosclerosis in their coronary arteries.

If you are a Type A person, you are probably tense and unable to relax. You work long and hard and eat and talk faster than many other people. You may have a strong sense of urgency about everything in your day-to-day life; you never have enough time. Your temper may be short, and you generally expect too much from your co-workers. You perceive yourself as being constantly under stress. On the other hand, if you are a Type B person, you are usually calm. You are not always speeding off somewhere, and you are not always feeling closed in by the pressures of life. However, even if your life is full of stresses and hardships, you are not automatically a Type A person. The key is in how you handle the stress. The Type B person handles stress better than the Type A person.

Even beyond Type A behavior, other psychological factors may play a role in physical health. Anxiety, depression, overwork, and social conflict may also increase susceptibility to hypertension and coronary artery disease.

Reducing Stress

Reducing stressful factors can contribute to lowering your blood pressure. To reduce stress, whenever possible, do things that relax you. Enjoy a hobby. Read. Write a letter to a friend or take a long walk. Activities that relax you, according to the

National Institutes of Health, "frequently break the cycle of too much adrenaline and allow the blood vessels to open up. Blood pressure will be lowered temporarily."

If you want to consider shifting your personality more from Type A to Type B, you might place more importance on what you do each day rather than on how much you do.

Many people have stressful factors in their work or family life that they cannot change. If you are one of these individuals, look at ways to change your manner of coping with these stresses. In many cases, adopting a more relaxed attitude can make a difference in the amount of stress you feel.

EFFECTS OF LIFESTYLE CHANGES

You can help yourself to health by finding ways to change your lifestyle according to your physician's recommendations. When you handle stress better, lose some weight, and exercise more, you may notice a reduction in your blood pressure. Coupled with a healthier diet, these changes can help you lead a healthier, more productive life.

If you smoke, quit smoking. (You read about the dangers of smoking in Chapter 4.) Exercise will be easier once you quit smoking, because your breathing capacity will begin to increase. In turn, you will be able to exercise more, to the point where you can achieve a training effect and strengthen your cardiovascular system.

For many people with hypertension, changes in lifestyle can mean the difference between needing and not needing medication to control their high blood pressure.

8

High Blood Pressure Medications

You are probably one of the 85 percent of all high blood pressure patients who can reduce and control their high blood pressure. According to the National Institutes of Health, this is true regardless of the severity of your hypertension. Some can do it with diet and weight reduction. Others require medication.

If you have been told that you require medication, be sure to follow your physician's recommendations carefully. Through a step-by-step procedure, and in a fairly short time, your physician will determine the optimal dose of a high blood pressure drug for you with minimal side effects. There is a major problem with high blood pressure medication: because hypertension is usually an asymptomatic disease (a disease that shows no symptoms), many patients do not feel a need to continue taking their medication. This is dangerous. Once they're off their medication, their blood pressure begins to go back up—and they may not know their blood pressure is again out of control.

While high blood pressure can be controlled, it is important to remember that there is no cure except in the cases of secondary hypertension for which a demonstrated underlying cause can be corrected. The drugs work only as long as you continue to take them. If you are advised to take medication for your hypertension, your physician's greatest concern is that you may neglect to take your medication.

Because all drugs have effects and side effects, and also interact with each other, it is important to tell your doctor if you are taking any other prescription drugs or over-the-counter medications when a high blood pressure medication is prescribed. You may also want to discuss the interaction of drugs you are taking with a pharmacist. Sometimes other drugs can counteract the effectiveness of your high blood pressure pills, and you should avoid such conflicts whenever possible.

THE MEDICATIONS

Your physician may prescribe one of many medications for you. Your prescription may be from one or more of the five major classes of high blood pressure drugs: diuretics, sympatholytics, vasodilators, beta blockers, and drugs that affect the central nervous system.

To understand how these drugs work it helps to realize that important elements of both your central and peripheral nervous systems are outside of consciousness and voluntary control, and automatically regulate many tissues such as glands, the heart, viscera, the iris of your eyes, and the muscles in the walls of your blood vessels. This system, the autonomic, is divided into two opposing parts—the sympathetic and the parasympathetic systems.

The sympathetic nervous system generally prepares your body for stressful situations, while the parasympathetic nervous system prepares your body for more sedentary activities. When you exercise, work hard, or worry excessively the sympathetic system is at work. It is the system responsible for constricting blood vessels and thus driving up your blood pressure in times of action or worry. When your nervous system prepares you for hard work or an emergency it speeds up your heart, constricts your blood vessels, and opens up the airways. These things increase your blood flow and make it easier to breathe. They ready your system for what scientists refer to as "fight or flight."

Thus, if a drug can decrease the activity of the sympathetic nervous system, it is easy to understand how it may lower your blood pressure.

The Diuretics

Your doctor may prescribe a diuretic for you. Diuretics are the most common high blood pressure medications. Most patients who have mild or moderate hypertension can be treated with these drugs alone. They act by increasing the kidney's excretion of sodium and reducing fluid retention. The drugs decrease the volume of fluid in the body and in the blood and in doing so lower the blood pressure. Because most patients tend to respond well to these drugs, they are usually the physician's first choice for medication.

The thiazide diuretics are the most frequently used diuretics. The thiazides were developed in the late 1950s from the sulfa compounds, which were used to fight off bacterial infections. The thiazides include drugs such as chlorothiazide and hydrochloro-thiazide. Another diuretic, chlorthalidone, is a thiazide derivative.

Sometimes effective diuretics lead to an undesirable reduction of potassium in the body, a disorder known as hypokalemia. Other drugs, such as spironolactone and triamterene, generally do not lead to hypokalemia and are therefore useful for controlling hypertension without this side effect. They are not, however, as effective as the thiazides.

Furosemide and ethacrynic acid are two other diuretics; both drugs are more potent than the thiazides. If you have kidney problems, however, your physician may prefer to prescribe these drugs for you.

Sympatholytics

Sympatholytic drugs reduce the action of the involuntary sympathetic nervous system, which, in preparing us for "fight or flight" emergencies, has a potent effect in sustaining and raising the blood pressure. They block transmission of the sympathetic nerve impulse. The classic sympatholytic drug is guanethidine. Normally, norepinephrine is responsible for carrying the message across the gap from the nerve to the muscle fibers in the blood vessel walls, causing the vessels to constrict. Guanethidine, though, acts to deplete stores of this chemical, limiting involuntary signals to the blood vessels to constrict. This permits dilation and thereby brings the blood pressure down.

Guanethidine is a very potent antihypertensive drug; usually it is used only for patients with severe hypertension. Its side effects may be more severe than those of other antihypertensive drugs; it often is prescribed under close supervision. It can cause hypotension (undesirably low blood pressure). In severe hypotension blood flow to the brain may be inadequate even to the point of fainting. Guanethidine may also cause a stuffy nose, diarrhea, or sexual dysfunction.

Beta Blockers

The beta blockers are multiple-action drugs that also influence a part of the sympathetic nervous system. They work by blocking the effects of stimulation coming to the heart and blood vessels through a special group of sympathetic nerve fibers called *beta adrenergic.* These drugs decrease cardiac output by acting on nerve receptor sites in the heart. In this way they decrease the amount of sympathetic nervous input into the heart—the heart rate slows, the heart does not work as hard, less blood is pumped, and blood pressure goes down. The beta blockers also suppress the system of hormones responsible for directly constricting blood vessels and retaining salt and water in the body.

Some beta blockers may cross into and accumulate in the brain, causing adverse central nervous system effects. Thus some beta blockers have been shown to cause depression and sleep disturbance. Beta blockers may have other side effects—they may aggravate bronchial asthma or cause fatigue, skin rashes, or hypotension.

The beta-blocking drugs include propranolol, atenolol, nadolol, metoprolol, and timolol.

One interesting side effect of the beta blockers is that shown by propranolol. The drug may limit your maximum heart rate, thus putting an upper limit on how intensely you can exercise before growing tired or simply not being able to move any faster. This is because the heart cannot supply the blood for the additional work. For this reason some athletes may not be able to perform to their limits if they are taking propranolol. In such cases the physician will recommend another drug. Drugs of this class should not be precipitously discontinued, but slowly tapered off over a period of one to two weeks or more if they are to be stopped or replaced by another type of medication.

Calcium Channel Blockers

In 1982 another class of drugs which inhibit blood vessel spasm became available for use in certain cardiac patients. The calcium blocking drugs inhibit the constriction of blood vessels. Drugs of this class may eventually be useful in helping some patients with hypertension.

Vasodilators

The vasodilators act directly to dilate the blood vessels. Once dilated, the vessels offer less resistance to blood flow and blood pressure is reduced.

The most common vasodilator is hydralazine. Other vasodilators include minoxidil and prazosin. Vasodilators are generally safe on a long-term basis when used under a physician's careful supervision.

It should be noted, however, that vasodilators may cause such side effects as headache, flushing, weakness, nausea, and chest pain.

Drugs That Affect the Central Nervous System

Some drugs act on the central nervous system and reduce the

action of the sympathetic nervous system by altering the chemical balance within the brain. Effects in the brain ultimately slow the heart rate and decrease the action in some nerves that control blood vessel constriction.

The most widely used drugs in this category at this time are methyldopa and clonidine. Clonidine may cause persistent drowsiness and dryness of the mouth. Physicians advise cutting down on such medications slowly when adverse effects occur. Suddenly cutting off this medication can trigger a sudden "overshoot" in your blood pressure, a rise that can be dangerous.

TRANQUILIZERS AND BIOFEEDBACK

Many people find that emotional stress and anxiety can raise their blood pressure. In these patients a tranquilizer may reduce their feelings of immediate tension. In most patients, however, a tranquilizer will not effectively lower the blood pressure. Tranquilizers are *not* high blood pressure drugs. Do not be fooled into thinking that because a tranquilizer helps you calm down and reduces psychological tension, your hypertension is also reduced. Remember, more often than not, hypertension has no symptoms. You can't really feel whether your pressure is high at any given time.

Some people think biofeedback helps to reduce blood pressure, but a recent National Heart, Lung, and Blood Institute study showed that some people achieved mild reductions in blood pressure during the biofeedback session, but what they learned was not effectively carried over between sessions, nor was it effective after the therapy was stopped. You might become interested in trying biofeedback, but if you do, be sure to continue using whatever medications are prescribed for you and adhering to appropriate diet and exercise habits.

HOW DOCTORS USE HYPERTENSION DRUGS

Your physician may follow a course of treatment for you known as *stepped care.* In the stepped care system your physician will advise you to begin with a thiazide diuretic, the drug most likely to benefit the average high blood pressure patient. If the diuretic is enough for you, your doctor will not prescribe other drugs right away. If it is not, he will move up to the next step. The second drug will be aimed at a different element of your problem. In this way, in sequential steps, your doctor will try different drugs until the effective drug or combination of drugs is found. Each patient is different because each combination of factors leading to high blood pressure is different. What works for one patient may not be effective for another.

TAKING YOUR HYPERTENSION DRUGS

Once your physician prescribes a high blood pressure medication for you, it is important that you take it according to directions. One of the most serious problems with the use of high blood pressure drugs is that too many patients misuse or neglect them. This can be dangerous. For example, forgetting to take a drug like clonidine could cause a life-threatening overshoot of blood pressure, as mentioned earlier.

Only about one in five among the millions of people in the United States and Canada who have prescriptions for antihypertension medications is taking enough medicine to do himself or herself any good. "Under traditional conditions of treatment more than 50 percent of hypertensive patients discontinue therapy entirely on their own within a year of starting it," Dr. David L. Sackett of the Department of Clinical Epidemiology, McMaster University, Hamilton, Ontario, reported recently.

Some patients may have to take as many as 10–15 pills a day; prescribing 2 or 3 is not uncommon. For this reason most physicians try to prescribe drugs that may be taken in one tablet, rather than several, a day. A single tablet does not necessarily have to contain only one drug—combination pills are often prescribed when appropriate.

If you experience any side effects from your medication, do not stop taking it; rather, let your doctor know about it right away. He or she will work with you to find another more suitable drug if the side effect is severe or persistent.

Your physician may want to teach you how to take your own

blood pressure at home. Doing so can save you money as well as waiting time in the physician's office. When you take your own blood pressure you can discuss your records with your physician during routine visits. You will learn more about monitoring your own blood pressure in the next chapter.

You can help your physician help you by integrating your medication into your daily habits. This way you are less likely to forget to take it. If this means taping your pills to your can of shaving cream, do so. Perhaps keeping your pills near your tube of toothpaste will remind you to take them each morning. Taking your medication regularly, as prescribed, is essential to proper control of your high blood pressure.

While your high blood pressure cannot be cured, it can be controlled with proper medication. In order for your medication to be effective, you must take it as your physician directs. The level of medication in your body must remain constant to ease the pressure on your blood vessels. Remember to refill your prescription before you use the last of your supply. Always refill your prescription before you leave on a trip so that you don't run out while away from home.

9

Self-Monitoring, Community Services, and Other Resources

Your physician and health care team will help you toward better health each time you visit their health center or office. They will make recommendations for alterations in your treatment plan that may include modifying your diet, increasing the amount of exercise you get, showing you better ways to cope with stress, and possibly reducing your medications.

Your health care team may also make other recommendations that go beyond these aspects. Additional advice might include suggestions to monitor your own blood pressure, participate in a community-based health care program, and read more about high blood pressure.

MONITORING YOUR OWN BLOOD PRESSURE

While some physicians recommend regular self-monitoring of blood pressure at home for some patients, there is some controversy among physicians regarding this procedure. The physicians who recommend it usually carefully select the patients for whom they recommend it. Some physicians say self-monitoring is particularly advisable for a group of people with what they call *borderline high blood pressure*. This means blood pressure that occasionally goes over the 90 mm Hg diastolic reading during visits to the office. Because the readings are different each time the patients are examined in the office, the physicians ask the patients to monitor their blood pressure daily at home to detect responses to therapy.

Ask your physician about the advisability of monitoring your own blood pressure at home between visits to the health center. You may be advised to monitor your pressure daily or several times a day during the early stages of your treatment until a well-balanced program of diet, exercise, and medication is established. After your program for controlling your high blood pressure seems to be working you may be advised to do your monitoring routine less frequently.

If your physician recommends that you take your blood pressure at home, you may be advised to get a moderately priced stethoscope and sphygmomanometer or a device with the stethoscope built right into the blood pressure cuff. Your physician will explain the various types of equipment available and what will best meet your needs. You can purchase these units at a drugstore, department store, medical supply outlet, or by mail order.

You can be trained by a nurse or other health care professional in about 20 minutes to take your own blood pressure. Your training will be successful if you can repeatedly report blood pressure readings within 5 mm Hg of the instructor's reading. Your physician will want to check your technique for self-monitoring after you have had your instruction and practiced with your own equipment a few times.

There are advantages and disadvantages to self-monitoring. Your health care team will explain how they relate to you as an individual.

The advantages include being able to take your own blood pressure at different times of the day to determine your average reading. You can avoid the tension you might feel in the physician's office by relaxing at home before you take your blood pressure. You can take it every day or several times a day if you are advised to do so, and report to your physician any changes you note. Another advantage is that the self-monitoring will serve as a reminder to you to take your medication, if you are on any, or to adhere closely to the diet and exercise routine your physician has recommended for you.

Disadvantages include becoming more nervous and tense about your blood pressure and consequently causing your pressure to go up even more. You can become so absorbed in taking your blood pressure that the issue becomes an even more important factor in your life than it should be. You may also have difficulty in reading the gauge and consequently report erroneous readings to your physician. Of course, your health care team will retake your blood pressure at each visit and will not depend entirely on your at-home reports for adding or changing medication but may find your readings helpful in evaluating your overall progress.

Many people find taking their blood pressure at home an easy part of their daily routine. Although the instructions that come with the self-monitoring devices explain in detail how to use them, the following explanation will give you a general idea of how you can use the basic stethoscope and blood pressure cuff combination.

Instructions may advise you to sit with your right arm resting at heart level on a tabletop with the inner side of your elbow and the palm of your hand facing upward. Next, apply the cuff smoothly about one or two inches above the bend of your elbow and apply the stethoscope head over a spot on your forearm where you can feel a strong pulse. Insert the earpieces of the stethoscope as instructed and then inflate the rubber bladder inside the blood pressure cuff by squeezing it repeatedly. This is the time to watch the dial on the measuring gauge. After the pressure within the bladder rises the dial will react slightly with each heartbeat. The thumping sounds you hear in the stethoscope are your heartbeats. Continue to inflate the cuff to about 20–30 mm Hg above the point where you hear no more sounds. Then, by slowly releasing air, you allow the pressure in the cuff to fall. The point at which you hear the first sound is your systolic pressure. Your instruction manual will show you exactly how to do this. As your pressure falls you will hear a louder sound with each heartbeat; the sounds first become louder and then fainter. The point at which you hear no more sounds is your diastolic pressure.

It is usually advisable to take your pressure a second time after a few minutes of relaxation and keep a record of both readings.

While self-monitoring devices are intended to be used by the person being tested, some people have difficulty in pumping up the cuff and releasing air from it while using their other hand to hold the stethoscope. Others have difficulty in hearing the sounds. If you experience any difficulties that may interfere with your efficiency in taking your own blood pressure, you may want someone else to assist you. However, that person should also receive appropriate instructions from your health care team.

Should others in your family use your equipment to take their blood pressures? Should everyone take their own blood pressure at home? Most physicians generally don't recommend that people whose blood pressure is within a normal range monitor their own pressure regularly. Such procedures, they say, may lead to hypochondria and overconcern about a nonexistent problem. Also, appropriate instruction and checking of the equipment is necessary to get accurate readings.

HELP FROM YOUR COMMUNITY

You may live in a community that provides valuable assistance to persons with high blood pressure. Some programs are supervised by community centers, health-related associations, or local boards of health. Many communities provide screening and monitoring programs for local residents. Screening programs usually involve measuring blood pressure in a large group of people and reporting results to the participants or their physicians for follow-up care. Many people are identified as having high blood pressure in a group screening program carried on at their place of work or in their community. Perhaps your high blood pressure was detected in that way.

One such community screening and monitoring program that has served as an example for many other American cities is that of the Department of Health in Skokie, Illinois, a suburban community of 60,000 people northwest of Chicago. The screening program began in the early 1970s and has since expanded to include a monitoring program. On certain days of the week blood pressure readings are taken by trained health professionals. Counseling is provided for those with high readings so that they will understand what having high blood pressure means. Diagnosis and treatment are not part of the service, however. Results are sent to the residents' doctors. Anyone who has no physician is given a list of local physicians. Once the people are under treatment they may return regularly to participate in the village's monitoring program for high blood pressure and have their pressure checked, without charge, by a health care professional. The information obtained during these monitoring sessions is sent directly to the physicians. This service saves residents the costs of visits to their doctors. The local doctors favor the system because it permits them to get a professionally taken blood pressure reading for patients at more frequent intervals than they could do in their offices. Some physicians prefer this routine to having patients monitor their own blood pressure at home or having it taken in drugstores, which may not always use accurate equipment.

In Skokie the Department of Health also brings its blood pressure detection and monitoring program to some of the residents. Each month a nurse and one volunteer visit a local housing complex for senior citizens and take blood pressures. Many new cases of high blood pressure are detected and referred for treatment this way.

To find out if your community has such a service and how it can serve you, contact your city, county, or state board of health or your local American Heart Association affiliate. Your physician and health care team will probably know if such a program exists and if it will be practical for you to have your blood pressure monitored regularly this way between visits to your health center.

Community-based preventive health care programs aimed at detecting and doing something about high blood pressure aren't just an American phenomenon. One outstanding example is in

Switzerland, where four towns participated in the Swiss National Research Program on primary prevention of cardiovascular disease between 1979 and 1981. The main question was: "Is it possible to convince a community to adopt a healthier lifestyle?" Results indicated that health education did convince people. At the beginning of the project residents in each of two test towns (where educational activities were planned) and two control towns (where no activities were planned) were tested for blood pressure, cholesterol level, smoking habits, and other lifestyle factors. At the end of the three-year period they were again tested for the same characteristics. At the end of the project period the proportion of people with known and controlled hypertension was substantially larger among the group screened at the start of the project than among an independent sample examined at the end of the project. The proportion of hypertensives controlled by treatment was larger in the test towns than in the control towns. This project, centered around Aarau (a German-speaking town) and Nyon (a French-speaking town) and their control counterparts, Solothurn and Vevey, indicated the importance of health screening and following through with educational programs planned for people identified as having high blood pressure. Participants attended classes, lectures, and demonstrations to learn how to control their own blood pressure. Activities involved groups under the guidance of a dietitian, nurse, or social worker in promoting blood pressure control through good eating habits, physical fitness, relaxation, and nonsmoking.

Participants in the diet education programs showed a significant reduction of blood cholesterol in comparison with a sample of nonparticipants matched by age, sex, and nationality. Participants in the test towns showed a smoking "quit rate" of about 26 percent as compared with a quit rate of 18 percent in the control towns. The proportions of nonsmokers who began to smoke during the same period was 5 percent in the test towns and 8 percent in the control towns.

Health education did make a difference, and it can make a difference for you. If your community offers health education classes, lectures, or programs, become a participant. If you pick up only one helpful hint during each program, you'll be that much ahead.

BOOKS ON HIGH BLOOD PRESSURE

While this book is intended as an introduction to, or a brief refresher course on, the fundamentals of high blood pressure, many other books are available that may interest you. Some are written for people with hypertension. Others are written for their families. The books are written at varying levels of complexity, and some concentrate on specific aspects of high blood pressure. Most are available at your local bookstore or public library, where you may enjoy browsing through the selection of books in the health section. Also, your health care team may recommend books that address your specific interests.

Books that you may find helpful include those listed below.

American Heart Association. *Heartbook: A Guide to Prevention and Treatment of Cardiovascular Diseases.* New York: E. P. Dutton, 1980.

This is a reference book about the major forms of diseases of the heart and blood vessels. It includes chapters on risk factors, stroke, hypertension, diet and nutrition, cholesterol, smoking, exercise, and how to live with heart disease.

Feinman, Max L., MD, and Wilson, Josleen. *Live Longer: Control Your Blood Pressure.* New York: Coward, McCann and Geoghegan, Inc., 1977.

This book explains high blood pressure and its relation to obesity, stress, and smoking and how high blood pressure can be controlled by diet, drugs, and changes in lifestyle.

Freis, Edward D., MD, and Kolata, Gina Bari. *High Blood Pressure Book: A Guide for Patients and Their Families.* New York: Painter Hopkins Publishers (a Division of Elsevier-Dutton Publishing), 1979.

This book provides information on the nature of hypertension and current treatments to control high blood pressure, including drugs and how they work, the effects of salt, altered lifestyles, diet, exercise, and biofeedback.

Lieberman, Ellin, MD. *Children Have Hypertension, Too! A Handbook for Pediatric Hypertension.* Los Angeles: American Heart Association, Greater Los Angeles Affiliate, 1979.

This book was developed under a grant made by the American Heart Association, Greater Los Angeles Affiliate. It discusses the recognition and control of hypertension in individuals less than 20 years of age.

Nutrition Task Force, American Heart Association, Texas Affiliate, Inc. *Children's Help Your Heart Cookbook.* Dallas: AHA/National Center, 1980.

This is a cookbook that was developed to encourage an awareness of good nutrition in elementary school youth. It gives the new cook safety tips, a table of measurements, information on how to measure, and a glossary of cooking terms. Recipes range from breakfast dishes to sweet treats and snacks.

Rees, Michael K., MD. *The Complete Family Guide to Living with High Blood Pressure.* Englewood Cliffs, NJ: Prentice-Hall, 1980.

This book provides a detailed discussion of high blood pressure, how it is measured, and why it must be controlled. It provides extensive information on available medications. Also included are chapters on ways to exercise, the pill, pregnancy, childhood hypertension, and blood pressure measurement at home.

Booklets and Miscellaneous Literature

Booklets are available from many authoritative sources. Some are free, and some require small payments in advance. Each source will also be able to guide you toward other sources for reading materials centered around your specific interests.

The High Blood Pressure Center of the National Institutes of Health provides many brochures and pamphlets. Topics include basic information about high blood pressure, dietary management of high blood pressure, and complications. Some are printed for

Hispanic readers. For a complete listing of available materials, write to:

High Blood Pressure Information Center
National High Blood Pressure Education Program
120/80 National Institutes of Health
Bethesda, MD 20205

The American Heart Association has many publications for which there is no charge or there is a nominal charge. Topics include facts about heart disease, high blood pressure, and what women should know about high blood pressure. Contact your local affiliate of the American Heart Association or write to:

American Heart Association
7320 Greenville Ave.
Dallas, TX 75231

The World Health Organization publishes many reports concerning the status of high blood pressure research, and its occurrence and treatment throughout the world. If you are interested in summaries of research efforts and current attitudes regarding treatment from many experts, you may want to write to the WHO:

World Health Organization
Distribution and Sales Service
1211 Geneva 27
Switzerland

Additionally, many publications about high blood pressure may be available without charge from reading racks at your physician's office or at your local health department.

By self-monitoring your blood pressure and taking advantage of health education programs in your community, you can become more informed about high blood pressure and how it is affecting you. This in turn will better prepare you to understand your health care team's instructions regarding your participation in controlling your high blood pressure.

10

Take Care of Yourself

You can help yourself to health while you and your physician work to control your blood pressure. You probably are taking more of an active interest in your health than you did before. Now that you know you have one of the risk factors for developing cardiovascular disease you probably are paying more attention to your diet, daily exercise habits, and rest and relaxation routines than you did before. If your high blood pressure has been detected at an early stage and you begin treating it right away, you may actually become healthier than you were before because of these important lifestyle changes.

YOUR DOCTOR: YOUR PARTNER

You and your doctor have formed a partnership regarding your health care. Each of you has a responsibility. Your doctor's part of the bargain is to give you the best possible advice to bring your high blood pressure under control. Your part is to follow instructions and carry out your individualized treatment plan. In addition to following your doctor's recommendations you will want to ask questions that will bring you to an even better mutual understanding. For example, if your doctor has just told you that you have high blood pressure, discuss the possibilities of trying to reduce it with lifestyle changes alone. Many people do. If you have been taking a blood pressure medication for a long time, discuss how you might be able to reduce the dosage of your medication by losing weight and exercising more.

If your physician strongly recommends medication for controlling your blood pressure, ask if your therapy is being initiated with a small dosage of an antihypertensive drug. Physicians often use a stepped care program, which means that you will be given an opportunity to control your blood pressure with a small dosage of medication, and the dosage of that drug will be increased or another drug will be added only after a sufficient time period has elapsed to determine the first drug's effect. The stepped care approach allows your physician to take advantage of the interaction of some drugs, which may mean that you can take smaller doses of individual drugs and minimize side effects.

If you notice any unfavorable side effects from your antihypertensive medication, discuss them with your physician. You may be able to switch successfully to another medication and avoid unpleasant reactions. Unless you describe exactly what you are noticing, your physician will not understand what experience you are having with your medication. While these drugs have been tested on large numbers of people, each person's reaction is slightly different.

If you are over age 65, for example, you may react to medications in ways that are different from the reactions of some younger people. Many older people are more sensitive to drugs than younger individuals. You will want to be completely honest with your physician in answering questions about your age, how you have reacted to other medications, and whether you are already taking some other medications.

While taking antihypertensive medications at any age, you will want to watch your sodium intake, weight control, and self-medications. Ask your physician before you take any medications for colds or allergies or any appetite suppressants. If you use any other medications, don't keep them secret.

When your physician recommends a treatment plan for your high blood pressure, with or without medication, you will want to have periodic checkups to find out how well you are controlling your disease. Ask how often you should return for examinations or if you should monitor your blood pressure elsewhere, such as at home or at a local community center. The frequency your doctor will recommend for your checkups may vary from a few weeks to several months, depending on the gradation of your high blood pressure and the general state of your health. If you are healthier and have fewer associated medical problems, you will be able to save money by requiring fewer visits.

MYTHS: DON'T BELIEVE THEM

Now that you know more about high blood pressure you will be aware of the prevalence of many myths about the disease. For example, some people may tell you that it's not necessary to take your high blood pressure medication to lower your blood pressure if you do the other things your doctor tells you to do. You may be trying to lose weight, cut down on use of salt, exercise more, and stop smoking. Some will say that, if you do all these things, taking the medication is not necessary. Don't listen. If your doctor prescribes regular medication for you, it is important to keep taking it while you follow the other recommendations.

Some think that having high blood pressure means that personal activities have to be cut down. Usually, controlling high blood pressure does not require a sedentary lifestyle or rest for improvement. On the contrary, exercise is often prescribed as part of the treatment for reducing and controlling high blood pressure.

You may have heard that people with high blood pressure get dizzy and have headaches. In some serious cases that's true, but not all people with high blood pressure have those symptoms, just as not all people with dizziness and headaches have high blood pressure. A person with high blood pressure can feel and look fine. Just because you feel and look well doesn't mean that your blood pressure is within a normal range. If you are given medication by your physician for reducing high blood pressure, continue taking it regularly, even if you have no symptoms.

When you tell some people that you have high blood pressure they may react with surprise because you usually seem to be calm. Some people think that having high blood pressure means being tense and anxious. Nervousness or tenseness does not necessarily lead to high blood pressure. Many even-tempered people have it. However, certain stresses may contribute to a rise in blood pressure, and continued stresses may have a long-term effect.

If you are over age 54 and have high blood pressure, you may think that it is normal because of your age. Hypertension is not necessarily a disease of older age. Many serious cases begin between ages 30 and 45 or earlier. Also, there once was a myth that blood pressure (at least the systolic reading) should be 100 plus the person's age. This is just a myth. If true, it would allow a 70-year-old to have a systolic reading of 170. With a blood pressure of 170/100 mm Hg his risk of future disease might be much greater than if his blood pressure were 120/90.

If, after a complete checkup by your doctor, you are told that you are fine but that you have "just a little high blood pressure, nothing to worry about," question your doctor more closely. Ask specifically what your blood pressure reading is. Ask if it is higher than it was the last time it was checked. Ask specifically if your diastolic reading is over 90 mm Hg. High blood pressure *is* something to worry about and to *do* something about. You might want to consider changing physicians and beginning a treatment plan. Untreated high blood pressure is the leading cause of strokes, heart disease, and kidney disease and the major contributor to about 100 deaths every day in the United States alone.

SOME STORIES YOU HEAR ARE TRUE

It is true that women with high blood pressure should not take oral contraceptives unless their physician specifically recommends them. Most physicians recommend other means of birth control for women with high blood pressure. If you are a sexually active female within childbearing age and have high blood pressure, discuss your needs for birth control techniques with your gynecologist. Be sure to say that you have high blood pressure.

It is also true that some women who never had high blood pressure before may develop it during pregnancy, because with the hormonal changes during pregnancy, there is a tendency to retain salt and water. For women who already have high blood pressure, pregnancy may cause the blood pressure to rise higher. In many cases the high blood pressure that develops during pregnancy may disappear after delivery. But if it continues, it is important to follow medical instructions carefully to control it.

What about men and women? Historically, men's chances of having high blood pressure have been greater than women's. This is no longer the case, especially after menopause. As women grow older, their chances of having high blood pressure are even greater than men's. Many women who had blood pressure within normal ranges during most of their lives find that their blood pressure is elevated after menopause. During and after this stage in a woman's life it is important to have blood pressure checked periodically.

It is also true that high blood pressure is more prevalent among black men and women than among white men and women. According to American Heart Association estimates, one of every three black Americans over age 18 has high blood pressure. If you are black, and particularly if you have a family history of high blood pressure or heart disease, it is important to have frequent checkups to be sure that your blood pressure is within normal limits. And, if it is elevated, begin treatment early, while it is still controllable by diet and exercise alone. Medication may be necessary for a short period of time. Do not delay treatment.

PRACTICAL ASPECTS: INSURANCE COSTS

In some cases life insurance premiums cost more for people with chronic conditions or major risk factors for cardiovascular disease. High blood pressure is one of these risk factors. Under some plans there may be limitations on coverage. Because there are many variations between individuals and insurance plans, if how your health relates to your insurance costs concerns you, discuss the matter with your insurance agent. Your general health will also be weighed in the decision about your acceptability as an insurance candidate. It will be to your continued advantage, for personal as well as monetary reasons, to keep your blood pressure under control and your overall health at optimum level.

Your health insurance may or may not pay for the costs involved in visiting your physician's office for routine checkups for your high blood pressure. You will want to look at your coverage to determine just what is and is not included. Does it cover repeated laboratory tests that may be necessary as part of your ongoing treatment? Some insurance plans cover diagnostic procedures, while others do not. Some cover expenses only after a certain deductible has been met. Health Maintenance Organizations (HMOs) may cover more of the costs of outpatient care and diagnostic tests with fewer deductibles than more traditional reimbursement or indemnity health insurance policies cover. Choose the system of health and medical care insurance that will provide you with the best-quality care within your range of choices and budget.

HELP YOURSELF TO HEALTH

This book has given you some basic guidelines with which you can help yourself to health. By carefully following your physician's instructions and asking questions about your treatment plan so that you fully understand the reasons behind the medical recommendations, you can take the most important steps toward health. Much of your treatment, however, will depend on your own participation. Your diet, weight control, exercise patterns, and mental outlook are your own responsibilities. So is your decision to smoke or not to smoke cigarettes.

Helping yourself to health means doing something good for those who care about you. By stopping smoking, if smoking has been your habit; choosing your foods wisely; cutting down on salt, cholesterol, and caloric foods; and building exercise into your daily routine, you can help those who love you worry less about your health.

If the person with high blood pressure is someone you love, help that person to better health by encouraging changes in lifestyle that will lead to healthful changes in blood pressure. Hugs and kisses are encouraging. Be supportive of the lifestyle changes. Encourage your loved one to follow the physician's orders.

Healthy people love life and are attractive to others. They are appealing as lovers, mates, co-workers, and friends. There is a spirit and sense of vitality that comes with good health that can't be replaced. Good health is your most precious possession. Guard it wisely. If your good health is threatened by high blood pressure, there are actions you can take to protect it. Start now to help yourself to health while you and your physician fight your high blood pressure.

Glossary

Adrenalin: The commercial name for a hormone secreted by the two small adrenal glands, which are just above the kidneys. Also called *epinephrine,* the secretion constricts the small blood vessels (arterioles), increases the rate of the heartbeat, and raises blood pressure.

Aldosterone: A hormone secreted by the adrenal cortex that promotes the conservation of salt and water by the kidneys.

Aneurysm: A ballooning-out of the wall of a vein, an artery, or the heart due to weakening of the wall by disease, traumatic injury, or an abnormality present at birth.

Angina pectoris: Acute pain in the chest resulting from decreased blood supply to the heart muscle. (The word *angina* is derived from the Greek word *anchone,* meaning strangling. *Pectoris* refers to the chest.) Angina pectoris may occur as a result of arteries narrowed by atherosclerosis or less commonly from spasm of the coronary arteries. Often the pain radiates from the heart to the shoulder, down the left arm, or into the neck and jaw.

Antihypertensive: Certain medications that are intended to lower high blood pressure.

Aorta: The main trunk artery that receives blood from the lower left chamber of the heart.

Arteriosclerosis: An older term referring to "hardening of the arteries"; the term covers a variety of conditions that cause the artery walls to thicken, lose elasticity, and reduce the flow of blood. (*See* atherosclerosis.)

Artery: A blood vessel that carries blood from the heart to various parts of the body.

Atherosclerosis: The preferred term for arteriosclerosis, in which the inner layers of the artery walls become thickened and irregular due to deposits of a fatty substance. The internal channel of the arteries become narrowed and the blood flow is reduced.

Atrium: One of the two upper chambers of the heart; sometimes also referred to as the *auricle*.

Beta blockers: Drugs that block the heart's response to stimulation of a part of the sympathetic nervous system. By regulating nerve impulses through the heart, beta blockers reduce heart rate, blood pressure, and the heart's oxygen requirements.

Blood pressure: The force or pressure exerted by the heart in pumping blood. The pressure of the blood against the walls of the arteries is determined by the pumping action of the heart, the elasticity of the walls of the main arteries, and the quantity of blood.

Calcium channel blockers: A class of drugs that inhibit blood vessel spasm and constriction of blood vessels. Eventually, they may be useful in helping some patients with hypertension.

Capillaries: The small blood vessels that carry oxygenated blood to all parts of the body.

Cardiac arrest: Occurs when the heart stops beating.

Cardiovascular: Pertaining to the blood vessels and the heart.

Cholesterol: A fatlike substance found mainly in meat, dairy products, and eggs. Dietary experts say that most Americans eat a diet containing too much cholesterol. They usually advise persons with high blood pressure or any other cardiovascular condition to reduce their cholesterol intake. Some people can eat liberal amounts of cholesterol and their serum cholesterol (their level of blood cholesterol) may not rise.

Congestive heart failure: A chronic condition (which can result from many diseases affecting the heart) in which the heart is unable to pump forcefully enough to deliver an adequate supply of blood throughout the body. Failure in the left ventricle can lead to pulmonary edema (fluid in the lungs), and failure of the right ventricle results in general edema with noticeable swelling in the hands and feet.

Coronary arteries: Two large arteries that branch from the aorta and supply the entire heart muscle with blood.

Diabetes mellitus: A disease in which the body is unable to utilize sugars properly, usually because the pancreas does not produce any insulin or does not produce enough insulin for the proper utilization of food to occur. It is often referred to as "diabetes."

Diastolic pressure: The blood pressure level during the relaxation phase between heartbeats. It is used as the primary indicator of hypertension. It is the lower reading when the blood pressure is recorded; for example, the 90 in 140/90 mm Hg.

Diuretics: Drugs that promote the excretion of urine. Diuretic drugs are prescribed chiefly to rid the body of excess fluid and sodium in high blood pressure or when it accumulates in tissues and causes edema (retention of water in the tissues of the body).

Edema: Swelling due to abnormally large amounts of fluid in the body tissues. Some causes include congestive heart failure and fluid and electrolyte imbalances, particularly those causing sodium retention.

Electrocardiogram: A test that graphically records and shows the electric currents produced by the heart; often called an ECG or EKG. Some abnormalities of heart function can be determined from the EKG.

Epinephrine: A hormone secreted by the adrenal glands. Another commercial name for it is *adrenalin.* One of its uses in the body is in constricting or squeezing arterioles and raising the blood pressure.

Heart attack: *See* myocardial infarction.

Hypertension or **high blood pressure:** Persistently high pressure of the blood against the arterial walls. *High* refers to higher than the normal range.

Hypotension: Blood pressure that is below the normal range.

Myocardial infarction: The medical term for *heart attack*; refers to death of the cells in an area of the heart muscle that has been deprived of oxygen and nutrients as a result of an obstruction in blood supply. The severity of a heart attack depends on which section of the heart it occurs in, and how extensively the muscle is damaged. If the infarction kills a part of the muscle that regulates the heart's electrical activity, the heartbeat may stop. The chances for recovery from many forms of heart attack are greatest with early and effective treatments.

Polyunsaturated fats: Fats that chemically can absorb additional hydrogen; usually liquid oils of vegetable origin such as corn and safflower oil. Dietary experts recommend that persons with high blood pressure or cardiovascular disease should include more fats that are polyunsaturated and fewer fats that are saturated in their daily diets.

Risk factors: The life habits that are thought to increase one's chances of developing cardiovascular disease. The most significant ones are high blood pressure, obesity, high cholesterol, and diabetes. Some experts also say that smoking cigarettes and consuming large quantities of alcohol and caffeinated beverages are also risk factors.

Saturated fats: Fats that chemically cannot absorb any more hydrogen. These are usually fats that are solid at room temperature and are of animal origin, such as fats in meat, milk, and butter. These are the fats the diet experts say should be restricted because they may lead to development of fatty deposits on the inside of the lining of the arteries and to atherosclerosis.

Sodium: An element that makes up nearly half the content of regular table salt; a mineral essential to life. Experts say its intake should be reduced to protect against cardiovascular disease and high blood pressure. In treatment of high blood pressure, reduction of sodium intake is usually strongly advised.

Stroke: Another term for cerebrovascular accident and apoplexy. It occurs when the blood supply to some part of the brain is impeded.

Sphygmomanometer: The most commonly used device to measure blood pressure.

Systolic blood pressure: The blood pressure inside the arteries when the heart contracts with each beat. It is the upper reading when the blood pressure is recorded; for example, the 140 in 140/90 mm Hg.

Vascular: Pertaining to blood vessels.

Ventricle: One of the two lower chambers (left and right) of the heart.

Index